PATIENT BILLING 7e

SUSAN M. SANDERSON

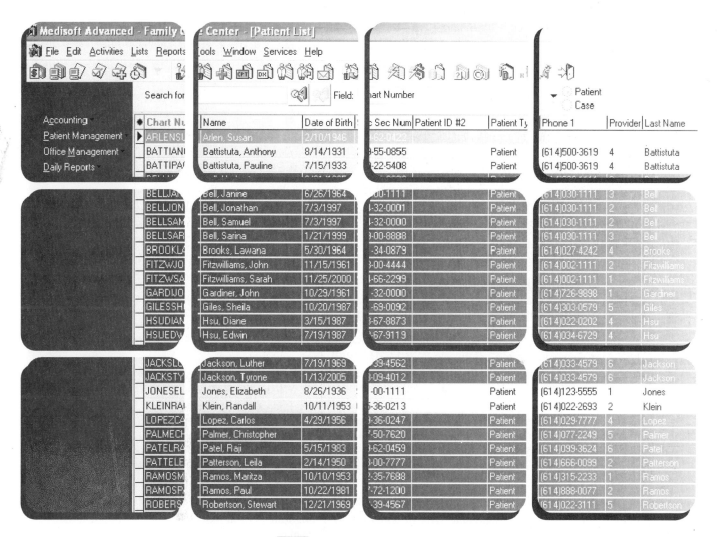

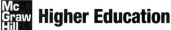 **Higher Education**

Boston   Burr Ridge, IL   Dubuque, IA   New York   San Francisco   St. Louis
Bangkok   Bogotá   Caracas   Kuala Lumpur   Lisbon   London   Madrid   Mexico City
Milan   Montreal   New Delhi   Santiago   Seoul   Singapore   Sydney   Taipei   Toronto

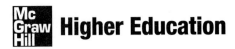

The McGraw-Hill Companies

Higher Education

PATIENT BILLING

Published by McGraw-Hill, a business unit of The McGraw-Hill Companies, Inc., 1221 Avenue of the Americas, New York, NY, 10020. Copyright © 2010 by The McGraw-Hill Companies, Inc. All rights reserved. Previous editions © 1989, 1995, 1998, 2003, 2006, and 2008. No part of this publication may be reproduced or distributed in any form or by any means, or stored in a database or retrieval system, without the prior written consent of The McGraw-Hill Companies, Inc., including, but not limited to, in any network or other electronic storage or transmission, or broadcast for distance learning.

Some ancillaries, including electronic and print components, may not be available to customers outside the United States.

 This book is printed on acid-free paper.

1 2 3 4 5 6 7 8 9 0 DOW/DOW 0 9

ISBN 978-0-07-340202-4
MHID 0-07-340202-8

Vice president/Editor in chief: *Elizabeth Haefele*
Vice president/Director of marketing: *John E. Biernat*
Sponsoring editor: *Natalie J. Ruffatto*
Director of development, Allied Health: *Patricia Hesse*
Freelance developmental editor: *Wendy Langerud,*
S4Carlisle Publishing Services
Executive marketing manager: *Roxan Kinsey*
Lead media producer: *Damian Moshak*
Media producer: *Marc Mattson*
Director, Editing/Design/Production: *Jess Ann Kosic*
Lead project manager: *Rick Hecker*

Senior production supervisor: *Janean A. Utley*
Designer: *Marianna Kinigakis*
Media project manager: *Mark A. S. Dierker*
Outside development house: *Susan Magovern,*
Chestnut Hill
Designer: *Marianna Kinigakis*
Cover designer: *Jessica M. Lazar*
Typeface: *11/13.5 Palatino*
Compositor: *Aptara®, Inc.*
Printer: *R. R. Donnelley*

Library of Congress Cataloging-in-Publication Data

Sanderson, Susan M.
    Patient billing / Susan M. Sanderson. — 7th ed.
        p. ; cm.
    Includes index.
    ISBN-13: 978-0-07-340202-4 (alk. paper)
    ISBN-10: 0-07-340202-8 (alk. paper)
    1. Medical fees—Computer programs—Handbooks, manuals, etc. 2. Collecting of
accounts—Computer programs—Handbooks, manuals, etc. I. Title.
    [DNLM: 1. Fees and Charges. 2. Office Automation. 3. Patient Credit and Collection.
4. Practice Management, Medical. 5. Software. W 74.1 S216p 2010]
    R728.5.S246 2010
    610.68'1—dc22

                                                                                            2008044952

The Medisoft Student Data files, illustrations, instructions, and exercises in PATIENT BILLING are compatible with the Medisoft™ Advanced Version 14 Patient Accounting software available at the time of publication. Adaptations may be necessary for use with subsequent versions of the software. Text changes will be made in reprints when possible. Medisoft Advanced Version 14 software must be available to access the Medisoft Student Data files. It can be obtained by contacting your McGraw-Hill sales representative.

All brand or product names are trademarks or registered trademarks of their respective companies.

CPT five-digit codes, nomenclature, and other data are copyright 2008 American Medical Association. All rights reserved. No fee schedules, basic unit, relative values, or related listings are included in the CPT. The AMA assumes no liability for the data contained herein.

CPT codes are based on CPT 2009

ICD-9-CM codes are based on ICD-9-CM 2009

All names, situations, and anecdotes are fictitious. They do not represent any person, event, or medical record.

www.mhhe.com

Brief Table of Contents

Contents

To the Student

Your Career in Medical Billing

This class introduces you to the concepts and skills you will need for a successful career in medical office billing. Health care continues to be one of the fastest growing industries. As such, there is increasing need for both health care professionals and support staff. One important support function involves the accounting and patient billing aspects of a medical practice. Individuals who have practical experience using patient billing software are well prepared for these challenging tasks. Anyone who aims to get a job in medical billing will find that an understanding of the billing cycle and billing software is often a prerequisite to being hired.

Billing specialists play important roles in the financial well-being of every health care business. Billing for services in health care is more complicated than in other industries. Government and private payers vary in payment for the same services, and healthcare providers deliver services to beneficiaries of several insurance companies at any one time. Medical billing specialists must be familiar with the rules and guidelines of each health care plan in order to submit the proper documentation so that the office receives maximum appropriate reimbursement for services provided. Without an effective billing staff, a medical office would have no cash flow!

To succeed in this field, you will need to possess a variety of abilities and skills. In addition to specialized knowledge about medical billing, you must have computer skills, including knowledge of database management, spreadsheets, electronic mail, and the Internet. You will also need to possess excellent customer service skills. Even though they are not involved in the actual process of providing medical care, billing specialists come in contact with clients, insurance companies, and patients. For example, incoming calls from patients who have questions regarding a charge are often directed to the billing staff, who must be able to communicate effectively with all types of people.

The position of medical billing specialist is one of the 10 fastest-growing occupations in allied health. This employment growth is the result of the increased medical needs of an aging population and the growing number of health practitioners. Medical billing is a challenging, interesting career, where you are compensated according to your level of skills and how effectively you put them to use. Those with the right combination of skills and abilities may have the opportunity to advance to management positions, such as patient account managers, physician office supervisors, and medical office managers. The more education the individual has, the more employment options and advancement opportunities are available.

About This Book

This text/workbook includes a tutorial and a comprehensive simulation. Once you learn how to operate the Medisoft program by completing the tutorial, you can practice those skills by working through the simulation. Both the tutorial and the simulation use a medical office setting, Family Care Center, to provide a realistic environment in which you can learn how to use the software.

Medisoft Advanced Patient Accounting is a popular patient billing and accounting software program. It enables health care practices to maintain their billing data as well as to generate report information. The software handles all the basic tasks that a medical billing assistant needs to effectively perform his/her job. As such, Medisoft is an excellent training tool for anyone interested in working as a medical billing assistant. Even if you do not use Medisoft on the job, the skills you learn here will be similar to those skills needed to use almost any medical accounting program. You will learn how to perform the following tasks:

- Input patient information
- Enter patient transactions
- Create insurance claims
- Produce patient statements
- Enter payments and adjustments
- Produce reports
- Enter patient appointments

The prerequisite for successful completion of *Patient Billing* is an understanding of the concepts and procedures for medical coding, billing, and reimbursement. This background can be obtained by studying McGraw-Hill's related insurance titles, the briefer, focused *From Patient to Payment* (Newby) or the longer, comprehensive *Medical Insurance* (Valerius/Bayes/Newby/Seggern). Students must also possess basic computer skills and familiarity with the Windows or Vista operating system.

After completing *Patient Billing*, students can build on their skills and enhance their qualifications for employment by studying *Case Studies for the Medical Office: Capstone Billing Simulation*, an excellent "internship in a box." *Case Studies for the Medical Office: Capstone Billing Simulation* contains a simulation covering two weeks of work in a medical office using Medisoft. In addition to providing activities through which students can practice and reinforce their basic Medisoft skills, the text/workbook introduces new Medisoft training topics that expand their knowledge.

Computer Supplies and Equipment

The Medisoft Student Data files for use with the exercises in *Patient Billing* are located at the text's Online Learning Center at *www.mhhe.com/patientbilling7e*. An Internet connection is required to download the files. The Medisoft Student Data files, which the author created for use with this textbook, provide a base of case study information. Other equipment and supplies needed are as follows:

- PC with 500 MHz or greater processor speed
- 256 MB RAM
- 500 MB available hard disk space (if saving data to hard drive)
- CD-ROM 2X or faster disk drive
- External storage device for storing backup copies of the working Medisoft Student Data files
- Windows Vista Business 32-bit version (Medisoft 14 will not work on the 64-bit system), Windows XP Professional, or Windows 2000 Professional
- Medisoft Advanced Patient Accounting, Version 14
- Printer

Getting Started

Before you jump into the tutorial, review the information provided in this section. Here you will find information that describes the setting and explains your role as a medical billing assistant at the Family Care Center.

Family Care Center

Dr. Katherine Yan, for whom you will work, operates the Family Care Center located in the Stephenson Medical Complex. This medical complex includes suites for 27 doctors, a pharmacy, and a laboratory with X-ray equipment. Like the other medical practices at the Stephenson Medical Complex, the Family Care Center is independently run. Referrals, however, are often made among the physicians in the complex.

Dr. Yan's Office Dr. Katherine Yan specializes in family practice, which means she is qualified to treat infants, children, and adults. She treats a wide variety of medical conditions, such as gynecological problems, cardiac problems, infections, and fractures. Dr. Yan is the first doctor her patients consult for almost any medical problem and for routine physical checkups as well. When patients need more specialized care, such as surgery or obstetrical services for the birth of a baby, Dr. Yan refers her patients to other doctors. Since a variety of specialists have offices in the complex, Dr. Yan is able to send most of her patients to other physicians there. In return, she sees patients who are referred to her by other doctors in the complex.

The office suite that Dr. Yan leases is located just off the landscaped courtyard in the center of the medical complex. Parking is nearby, providing easy access to the office for the physically handicapped patients. The office suite consists of the following rooms:

- A reception area with comfortable furniture and reading materials for adults and children. The office receptionist sits at a workstation in this area. Patients check in here when they arrive and make appointments and pay bills here when they leave. This is where the main office phone is located. The appointment scheduler is easily accessible so that the receptionist can schedule appointments when patients call the office.

- A spacious office off the reception area with a desk for the medical billing assistant, a computer, a variety of office equipment, and a wall of file drawers. Patient charts, patient financial and medical records, and other records are stored in this area. There is a phone in this area as well, so that the medical billing assistant can handle inquiries from patients and phone calls to patients and insurance companies about their bills and unpaid claims.

- An office for the office manager, next to the medical billing assistant's office.

- An adjacent hallway leading to the following rooms within the office suite: a minor surgery room, three examination rooms, a small laboratory for routine tests (other tests are performed at the laboratory in the medical complex), an office where Dr. Yan speaks with patients, a supply room with medical and office supplies, and a rest room.

The office is open Monday through Friday from 8:00 A.M. to 5:00 P.M. and on some Saturdays. Dr. Yan shares nonoffice-hour calls with six other doctors in the area. She is on call Tuesday evenings and every seventh weekend for emergencies. When Dr. Yan is on call, the members of her staff are also asked to be available in case they are needed.

Members of Dr. Yan's staff include:

- Doris Blackwell—Office Manager. Doris has been with the doctor for the past four years and supervises the business aspects of the practice. She also serves as the accountant for the office, doing payroll, accounts payable, and so on, working closely with a certified public accountant.

- Michelle Walcott—Clinical Assistant. Michelle has worked with Dr. Yan for the past six years. She prepares patients to see the doctor, gives injections, changes dressings, assists in minor surgery, and generally helps the doctor with patient care.

- David Gerardo—Receptionist/Administrative Medical Office Assistant. David handles the front desk and the phones, pulls patients' charts for daily appointments, files the charts, schedules appointments, and orders supplies.

- You—Medical Billing Assistant. Dr. Yan has recently hired you as the new medical billing assistant to replace Bill Larson, who has moved out of the area. Your first responsibility is to learn the

Medisoft patient billing and accounting software. Although your primary responsibility is for patient records and patient billing, Dr. Yan wants to be sure that you are familiar with the basic accounting system used in the office. The office uses the cash basis for accounting, which means that all revenues are recorded when they are actually received and that expenses are recorded only when they are paid. The patient billing portion of the accounting system has been computerized using Medisoft Advanced Patient Accounting.

Your Role   Since one of your major responsibilities is to handle patient accounts in Medisoft, Dr. Yan has asked that you become familiar with Medisoft as soon as possible. You will begin your training by reading materials about how a medical office operates and about how a computerized patient billing system works. The materials will enable you to learn and practice using the various functions of the software before you work with real information.

After you have completed Chapters 1 through 7 of the instructional materials, you will enter patient information for Dr. Yan's office for a four-day period. This will give you an opportunity to work with actual patient information and to try out what you have learned. The Appendix provides you with an opportunity to learn how to enter appointments in a medical practice using Office Hours, a program from the makers of Medisoft.

How Can I Succeed In This Class?

If you're reading this, you're on the right track.

"You are the same today that you are going to be five years from now except for two things: the people with whom you associate and the books you read." Charles Jones

Right now, you're probably leafing through this book feeling just a little overwhelmed. You're trying to juggle several other classes (which probably are equally as intimidating), possibly a job, and on top of it all, a life.

It's true—you are what you put into your studies. You have a lot of time and money invested in your education. Don't blow it now by only putting in half of the effort this class requires. Succeeding in this class (and life) requires:

- A commitment—of time and perseverance

- Knowing and motivating yourself

- Getting organized

- Managing your time

This special introduction has been designed specifically to help you learn how to be effective in these areas, as well as offer guidance in:

- Getting the most out of your lecture

- Thinking through—and applying—the material

- Getting the most out of your textbook
- Finding extra help when you need it

A Commitment—Of Time and Perseverance

Learning—and mastering—takes time. And patience. Nothing worthwhile comes easily. Be committed to your studies and you will reap the benefits in the long run.

Consider this: your accounting courses are building the foundation for your future—a future in your chosen profession. Sloppy and hurried craftsmanship now will only lead to ruins later.

Side note: A good rule of thumb is to allow 2 hours of study time for every hour you spend in lecture.

Knowing and Motivating Yourself

What type of a learner are you? When are you most productive? Know yourself and your limits and work within them. Know how to motivate yourself to give your all to your studies and achieve your goals. Quite bluntly, you are the one that benefits most from your success. If you lack self-motivation and drive, you are the first person that suffers.

Knowing yourself—There are many types of learners, and no right or wrong way of learning. Which category do you fall into?

- **Visual learner**—You respond best to "seeing" processes and information. Particularly focus on the text's figures and tables.

- **Auditory learner**—You work best by listening to—and possibly tape recording—the lecture and by talking information through with a study partner.

- **Tactile/Kinesthetic Learner**—You learn best by being "hands on." You'll benefit by applying what you've learned during lab time. Think of ways to apply your critical thinking skills in application ways. Perhaps a text website will also help you.

Identify your own personal preferences for learning and seek out the resources that will best help you with your studies. Also, learn by recognizing your weaknesses and try to compensate/work to improve them.

Getting Organized

It's simple, yet it's fundamental. It seems the more organized you are, the easier things come. Take the time before your course begins to look around and analyze your life and your study habits. Get organized now and you'll find you have a little more time—and a lot less stress.

- **Find a calendar system that works for you.** The best kind is one that you can take with you everywhere. To be truly organized, you should integrate all aspects of your life into this one calendar—school, work, leisure. Some people also find it helpful to have an additional monthly calendar posted by their desk for "at a glance" dates and to have a visual of what's to come. If you do this, be sure you are consistently synchronizing both calendars as not to miss anything. *More tips for organizing your calendar can be found in the time management discussion that follows.*

- **Keep everything for your course or courses in one place**—and at your fingertips. A three-ring binder works well because it allows you to add or organize handouts and notes from class in any order you prefer. Incorporating your own custom tabs helps you flip to exactly what you need at a moment's notice.

- **Find your space.** Find a place that helps you be organized and focused. If it's your desk in your dorm room or in your home, keep it clean. Clutter adds confusion, stress, and wastes time. Or perhaps your "space" is at the library. If that's the case, keep a backpack or bag that's fully stocked with what you might need—your text, binder or notes, pens, highlighters, Post-its, phone numbers of study partners (hint: a good place to keep phone numbers is in your "one place for everything calendar").

A Helpful Hint—add extra "padding" into your deadlines to yourself. If you have an assignment due on Friday, set a goal for yourself to have it done on Wednesday. Then, take time on Thursday to look over your work again, with a fresh eye. Make any corrections or enhancements and have it ready to turn in on Friday.

Managing Your Time

Managing your time is the single most important thing you can do to help yourself. And, it's probably one of the most difficult tasks to successfully master.

You are taking this course because you want to succeed in life. You are preparing for a career. You are expected to work much harder and to learn much more than you ever have before. To be successful you need to invest in your education with a commitment of time.

How Time Slips Away

People tend to let an enormous amount of time slip away from them, mainly in three ways:

1. **procrastination,** putting off chores simply because we don't feel in the mood to do them right away

2. **distraction,** getting sidetracked by the endless variety of other things that seem easier or more fun to do, often not realizing how much time they eat up

3. **underestimating the value of small bits of time,** thinking it's not worth doing any work because we have something else to do or somewhere else to be in 20 minutes or so.

We all lead busy lives. But we all make choices as to how we spend our time. Choose wisely and make the most of every minute you have by implementing these tips.

Know Yourself and When You'll Be Able to Study Most Efficiently

When are you most productive? Are you a late nighter? Or an early bird? Plan to study when you are most alert and can have uninterrupted segments. This could include a quick 5-minute review before class or a one-hour problem solving study session with a friend.

Create a Set Study Time for Yourself Daily

Having a set schedule for yourself helps you commit to studying, and helps you plan instead of cram. Find—and use—a planner that is small enough that you can take with you—everywhere. This can be a $2.50 paper calendar or a more expensive electronic version. They all work on the same premise—**organize** *all* **of your activities in one place.**

Less is more. Schedule study time using shorter, focused blocks with small breaks. Doing this offers two benefits:

1. You will be less fatigued and gain more from your effort, and

2. Studying will seem less overwhelming and you will be less likely to procrastinate.

Plan Time for Leisure, Friends, Exercise, and Sleep

Studying should be your main focus, but you need to balance your time—and your life.

Try to complete tasks ahead of schedule. This will give you a chance to carefully review your work before you hand it in (instead of at 1 A.M. when you are half awake). You'll feel less stressed in the end.

Prioritize!

In your calendar or planner, highlight or number key projects; do them first, and then cross them off when you've completed them. Give yourself a pat on the back for getting them done!

Try to resist distractions by setting and sticking to a designated study time (remember your commitment and perseverance!). Distractions may include friends and surfing the Internet. . . .

Multitask When Possible

You may find a lot of extra time you didn't think you had. Review material or organize your term paper in your head while walking to class, doing laundry, or during "mental down time." (Note—mental down time does NOT mean in the middle of lecture.)

Getting the Most Out of Lectures

Believe it or not, instructors want you to succeed. They put a lot of effort into helping you learn and preparing their lectures. Attending class is one of the simplest, most valuable things you can do to help yourself. But it doesn't end there . . . getting the most out of your lectures means being organized. Here's how:

Prepare Before You Go To Class

Really! You'll be amazed at how much more comprehensible the material will be when you preview the chapter before you go to class. Don't feel overwhelmed by this already. One tip that may help you—plan to arrive to class 5-15 minutes before lecture. Bring your text with you and skim the chapter before lecture begins. This will at the very least give you an overview of what may be discussed.

Be a Good Listener

Most people think they are good listeners, but few really are. Are you? Obvious, but important points to remember:

- You can't listen if you are talking.

- You aren't listening if you are daydreaming.

- Listening and comprehending are two different things. If you don't understand something your instructor is saying, ask a question or jot a note and visit the instructor after hours. Don't feel dumb or intimidated; you probably aren't the only person who "doesn't get it."

Take Good Notes

- Use a standard size notebook, and better yet, a three-ring binder with loose leaf notepaper. The binder will allow you to organize and integrate your notes and handouts, integrate easy-to-reference tabs, etc.

- Use a standard black or blue ink pen to take your initial notes. You can annotate later using a pencil, which can be erased if need be.

- Start a new page with each lecture or note taking session (yes—you can and should also take notes from your textbook).

- Label each page with the date and a heading for each day.

- Focus on main points and try to use an outline format to take notes to capture key ideas and organize sub-points.

- Review and edit your notes shortly after class—at least within 24 hours—to make sure they make sense and that you've recorded core thoughts. You may also want to compare your notes with a study partner later to make sure neither of you have missed anything.

Get a Study Partner

Having a study partner has so many benefits. First, he/she can help you keep your commitment to this class. By having set study dates, you can combine study and social time, and maybe even make it fun! In addition, you now have two sets of eyes and ears and two minds to help digest the information from lecture and from the text. Talk through concepts, compare notes, and quiz each other.

An obvious note: Don't take advantage of your study partner by skipping class or skipping study dates. You obviously won't have a study partner—or a friend—much longer if it's not a mutually beneficial arrangement!

Helpful hint: Take your text to lecture, and keep it open to the topics being discussed. You can take brief notes in your textbook margin or reference textbook pages in your notebook to help you study later.

Getting the Most Out of Your Textbook

McGraw-Hill and the author of this book, Susan, have invested our time, research, and talents to help you succeed as well. Our goal is to make learning—for you—easier.

Here's how:

Patient Billing includes many special features designed to help you master the Medisoft billing software. The major features are the following:

The text/workbook is divided into two separate sections—tutorial and simulation. The tutorial lets you learn the basic Medisoft software features, and the simulation helps you master the program. The tutorial thoroughly describes all of the Medisoft options and features that relate to patient billing.

To help you understand these new concepts, the tutorial uses the Family Care Center as a realistic medical office setting in which you perform many of the tasks. Step-by-step instructions guide you through each new activity. Practice exercises begin with simple tasks and progress to more complex activities throughout the tutorial. Before you complete the exercises, you must install the Medisoft Student Data files that were created for use with the text/workbook. Check with your instructor to determine whether these files have already been loaded on your computer. If your instructor has not already loaded the data, go to the Online Learning Center at *www.mhhe.com/patientbilling7e,* and follow the instructions for downloading the Medisoft Student Data.

The tutorial includes many screen illustrations, source documents, and sample reports to reinforce the concepts introduced in the text/workbook. Reminders or tips are placed throughout the tutorial. These tips identify shortcuts and list other helpful information for using the Medisoft program more effectively.

As you work through a chapter, follow these steps:

- Read the text. Study the figures and screen illustrations that accompany the explanations of various topics.

- As you read, answer the Checkpoint questions that appear throughout the chapter. Write your answers in the text/workbook. Look back at the text if necessary to determine your answer.

- Throughout the tutorial, there are practice exercises that you must complete at the computer. Work through each practice exercise by following the step-by-step instructions.

- Do not skip any practice exercises. You must complete all of the exercises before you begin the simulation.

- The source documents referred to in the practice exercises are located at the back of the book beginning on page 183.

- If you experience difficulty completing a practice exercise, review the corresponding section in the tutorial and then try the exercise again.

- Complete the chapter review questions after you finish each chapter.

When you have finished Chapters 1 to 7, complete the Patient Billing Simulation by following the instructions beginning on page 163 of the text/workbook. The simulation lets you step into the role of billing assistant for the Family Care Center and apply what you learned in the tutorial to the day-to-day activities of a medical practice. This also provides you with hands-on experience you can take with you into the job market!

To The Instructor

Patient Billing provides your students with the opportunity to learn and perform the duties of a medical billing assistant using Medisoft™ Advanced Version 14 Patient Accounting, a computerized patient accounting program. Medisoft™ Advanced Version 14 is available to schools adopting *Patient Billing*. Contact your McGraw-Hill sales representative for information on ordering and installing the software. You may also refer to the Instructor's Manual that accompanies the text. Student-at-Home Medisoft Advanced Version 14 is available as an option for distance education or for students who want to practice with the software at home.

Teaching students how to use a software application such as Medisoft can be a challenging endeavor. For this reason, this text/workbook is accompanied by several teaching and learning supplements.

Teaching and Learning Supplements

For the Instructor

Instructor's Software Medisoft™ Advanced Version 14 CD-ROM This full working version allows a school to place the live software on the laboratory or classroom machines (only one copy needs to be sent per campus location).

Instructor's Manual includes:

- Information on ordering and getting started with Medisoft™ Advanced Version 14 software

- Software troubleshooting tips and technical support

- Chapter-by-chapter teaching suggestions, checkpoint answers, end-of-chapter solutions, and sample printouts corresponding to the practice exercises

- Numerous printouts and solutions for the simulation so that you can check your students' work every step of the way or after they have finished the simulation

- Correlation tables: SCANS, AAMA Role Delineation Study Areas of Competence (2003), and AMT Registered Medical Assistant Certification Exam Topics

After you install the software and are ready for your students to begin using the Medisoft™ Advanced Version 14 program, you can rely on the manual for important information that will help your students work through the exercises in the book.

Online Learning Center (OLC), *www.mhhe.com/patientbilling7e,* Instructor Resources include:

- Instructor's Manual in Word and PDF formats

- Electronic testing program featuring McGraw-Hill's EZ Test. This flexible and easy-to-use program allows instructors to create tests from book specific items. It accommodates a wide range of question types and instructors may add their own questions. Multiple versions of the test can be created and any test can be exported for use with course management systems such as WebCT, Blackboard, or PageOut.

- PowerPoint® files for each chapter

- Health Insurance Claim Form (CMS-1500)

- End-of-chapter Medisoft backup files for Chapters 3–7, the Simulation, and the Appendix. These backup files can be used to help teachers evaluate students' work at the end of each chapter. By restoring the backup file for a given chapter, the instructor has easy access to the current state of the database when the exercises for that chapter have been completed. The backup files can also be provided to students who misplace or damage their Medisoft working data file during the course of the semester.

- Medisoft tips and frequently asked questions

- Medisoft™ Advanced Version 14 order and installation instructions

- Medisoft Student Data files (contain database to be used with exercises in the book); these files may be downloaded by the instructor or the students

- PageOut link

For the Student

Student-at-Home Medisoft Advanced Version 14. This version is an option for distance education or students who want to practice with the software at home.

Medisoft Student Data Files are available for download from the Online Learning Center, *www.mhhe.com/patientbilling7e.* The data files provide the patient database to complete the Medisoft™ Advanced Version 14 exercises in the text/workbook.

Online Learning Center (OLC), *www.mhhe.com/patientbilling7e.* In addition to information on downloading the Medisoft Student Data files, the site includes additional chapter quizzes, flash cards, and installation instructions for Medisoft Advanced Version 14 at-home software.

Acknowledgments

For insightful reviews, criticisms, helpful suggestions, and information, we would like to acknowledge the following individuals:

Reviewers of the Seventh Edition

CJ Bersani, AAS
Morrisville State College

Jennifer Bille
Tri-State Business Institute

Karen Coffey, MS Ed
University at Buffalo Educational Opportunity Center

Suzanne Cook-Turner, AA
Shoreline Workforce Development Services

Jennifer M. Evans, MA
South Seattle Community College

Rashmi Gaonkar, MS
ASA Institute

Yolande Beasley Gardner, MA
Lawson State Community College

Terri Harp, BS
Gordon Cooper Technology Center

Janet Hunter, MS, MBA, PhD
Northland Pioneer College

Christine Sproles, RN, BSN, MS
Pensacola Christian College

Mary Margaret Zulaybar
ASA Institute

Reviewers of the Sixth Edition

Melissa S. Cruz
Seacoast Career Schools

Barbara Desch LVN CPC AHI
San Joaquin Valley College

Shirley Eittreim-Shaw
Northland Pioneer College

Randi Haight, CPC
Sanford Brown Institute

Carol L. Jarrell, MLT,AHI
Brown Mackie College-Merrillville

Pat G. Moeck, PhD, MBA, BA, CMA
El Centro College

Jim Wallace, MHSA
Maric College

Reviewers of the Fifth Edition

Roxane Abbott
Sarasota County Technical Institute

Emil Asdurian, M.D.
Plaza College

Marcia Banks
The Chubb Institute, Olympia College

Yolanda Beasley Gardner
Bessemer State Technology Institute

Shawna Benton Harwell
Virginia College

Marion Bucci
Delaware Technical Community College

Margaret Dutcher
Virginia College

Christine Enz, MEd., CCS-P
Rochester Business Institute

George Fakhoury
Heald College

Marilyn Graham
Moore Norman Technology Center

Jodee Gratiot, CCA
Rocky Mountain Business Academy

Toni Hartley
Laurel Business Institute

Lisa Hauschild
Ivy Tech State College—Northeast

Cynthia R. Johnson, MLT (ASCP), LMT
Cleveland Institute of Dental Technology

Timothy P. MacDonald
Southern Maine Community College

Loreen W. MacNichol, CMRS, RMC
Andover College

Mary Jane Montgomery
ETI Technical College

Sherry L. Mulhollen, CMA, BS
Elmira Business Institute

Deborah Mullen
Sanford Brown Institute

Scott A. Norman
Bohecker College

Cindy L. Rosburg
Wisconsin Indianhead Technical Institute (WITC)

Lisa Smith-Proffitt
Hagerstown Community College

Deja Sprague
Regional Education Specialist Premier Education Group

Geiselle Thompson
The Learning Curve Plus

Jim Wallace
Maric College

Denise E. Wallen
Academy of Professional Careers

Danny Webb
Golden State College

Linda S. Weldon, CMA
Bryman College

Stacey F. Wilson, MT/PBT (ASCP), CMA
Cabarrus College of Health Sciences

Veronica J. Wright, BS, CPC
Concorde Career College

Cynthia Zumbrun, RHIT
Allegany College of Maryland

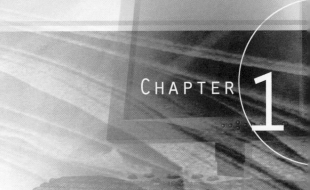

Introduction to Patient Billing

WHAT YOU WILL LEARN

When you finish this chapter, you will be able to complete the following objectives:

1-1. Define the terms introduced in this chapter.

1-2. Explain how patient billing fits into the overall accounting system.

1-3. List the ten steps in the medical billing process.

1-4. Define the financial records a medical billing assistant maintains.

1-5. Describe the data files maintained in a medical billing database.

1-6. Compare a manual patient billing system with a computerized system.

KEY TERMS

Accounting cycle The flow of financial transactions in a business.

Accounts receivable (AR) Monies that are coming into the business.

Case A grouping of procedures or transactions generally organized by the type of treatment or insurance carrier.

Cash payments journal Record of all cash payments, frequently in the form of a checkbook register.

Cash receipts journal Record of all cash received by a business.

CHAMPVA A government health insurance plan for disabled veterans.

CMS-1500 A paper insurance form accepted by government insurance plans in some states and by most private insurers (formerly HCFA-1500).

Consumer-driven health plan (CDHP) A plan in which a high-deductible/low-premium insurance plan is combined with a pretax savings account to cover out-of-pocket medical expenses.

CPT-4 Listing of codes for medical services or procedures.

Database A collection of information (data) arranged logically so that it can be stored and retrieved.

Data file A subset of data that is part of a larger database.

Day sheet Daily record of activities, patients treated, fees charged, and payments received.

Diagnosis The physician's determination of what is wrong with the patient, based on an examination.

Encounter form Record of one patient's visit showing procedures performed, charges, and diagnosis. In a manual system, this document may also be referred to as a fee slip, routing slip, or superbill.

General ledger Record of all the accounts of a business.

Guarantor The person or third party responsible for payment of a patient's medical bills.

HIPAA Security Rule Legislation that outlines the required administrative, technical, and physical safeguards to prevent unauthorized access to protected health care information.

ICD-9-CM Listing of codes for medical diagnoses; will eventually be replaced by ICD-10-CM.

Journal Record of daily transactions listed in chronological order, also known as the book of original entry.

Ledger A group of accounts in which debits and credits are posted from the book of original entry.

Medicaid Health insurance offered by the government for low-income people (called MediCal in California).

Medicare Government health insurance made available to elderly and disabled people.

Patient ledger Record of all activity (charges, payments, and adjustments) in an individual patient's account.

Procedure A service performed by a physician or other provider.

Providers The medical staff members, such as doctors and physical therapists, who perform the various services.

Real-time claims adjudication (RTCA) The submission and settling of an electronic health insurance claim at the time a patient checks out.

Transactions Charges, payments, and adjustments for services provided to patients.

TRICARE A government health insurance plan for eligible dependents of military personnel.

Overview of Medical Office Accounting

Like other businesses, a medical office must track the flow of money into and out of the practice. Keeping accurate financial records helps **providers**—the medical personnel who perform the various procedures—make sure that they are properly compensated for the services they perform. Financial data are also important for tax-reporting purposes and are useful in determining whether a practice is profitable.

Medical offices record their financial records in a series of journals and ledgers. A **journal** is a record of the daily transactions listed in chronological order, and a **ledger** shows the activity for each account. The **cash payments journal** lists payments made by check to vendors and employees; and the **cash receipts journal** is used to record any money received. To maintain these records, the billing assistant may use computers and patient billing and accounting software programs or may manually enter the data into books and accounting journals. For smaller offices with one or two practitioners, a combination of computer and manual systems is often used. Larger group practices that have full-time bookkeepers or office managers are more commonly computerized.

Patient billing, which involves tracking how much money patients owe and what they have paid, is a key part of a medical office accounting system. The patient billing duties are the primary responsibility of the medical billing assistant. Medical billing assistants maintain records, enter payments, update patients' ledgers, prepare patients' statements, and process insurance claims.

The **day sheet** (or general journal or daily journal) is a chronological record of all transactions involving patients. From the day sheet, information on the activity in each patient's account can be transferred to the appropriate patient ledger.

Once the billing assistant generates the patient ledgers, the accountant can use this information to update the general ledger. The **general ledger** includes up-to-date balances for all of a medical practice's accounts, and it is used to prepare various financial statements, such as income statements and balance sheets.

Day-to-Day Activities

As a billing assistant, your job is to follow a routine each day to keep the patient accounts up to date. These tasks are part of the medical billing process. The billing process consists of ten steps that lead to maximum, appropriate, timely payment for patients' medical services (see Figure 1-1 on page 4). As a billing assistant, you will have responsibilities associated with several of these steps.

The medical billing steps are as follows:

1. Preregister patients
2. Establish financial responsibility
3. Check in patients
4. Check out patients
5. Review coding compliance
6. Check billing compliance
7. Prepare and transmit claims
8. Monitor payer adjudication
9. Generate patient statements
10. Follow up payments and collections

Step 1 Preregister Patients

The first step in the billing and reimbursement process is to collect patient information. Part of this work is done in advance over the telephone; the other part is done when the patient arrives for an appointment.

Medical Billing Process

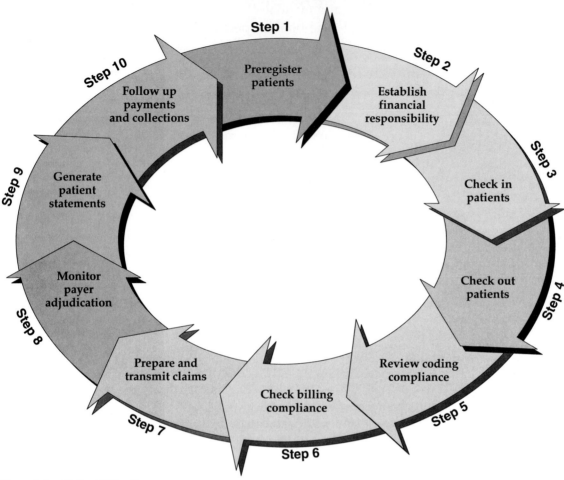

Figure 1-1 *Medical Billing Process*

Step 2 Establish Financial Responsibility

During the initial telephone call, it is important to ask whether the patient has insurance and, if so, to find out the specific type of coverage. Physicians usually participate in some insurance plans and not others; this information must be provided to the patient before the office visit, since it will affect the amount the patient will pay. For example, if the physician does not participate in an insurance plan, the patient may be liable for all charges.

Step 3 Check In Patients

When a new patient comes to the office for the first time, he or she fills out a patient information form that asks for his or her name, address, employer, insurance coverage, marital status, and so on (see Figure 1-2). When a patient moves, changes jobs, changes insurance carriers, or has other new information, that information must be entered on a patient information form as well. As the medical billing assistant, you must make sure that new and updated information is used in preparing insurance

PATIENT INFORMATION FORM

THIS SECTION REFERS TO PATIENT ONLY

Name: Lisa Lomos	Sex: F	Marital Status: [X]S []M []D []W	Birth Date: 6/3/04

Address: 12 Briar Lane	SS#: 212-55-3311		

City: Stephenson	State: OH	Zip: 60089	Employer:

Home Phone: 614-221-0202	Employer's Address:		

Work Phone: 614-299-0313	City:	State:	Zip:

Spouse's Name:	Spouse's Employer:

Emergency Contact:	Relationship:	Phone #:

FILL IN IF PATIENT IS A MINOR

Parent/Guardian's Name: Juan Lomos	Sex: M	Marital Status: []S [X]M []D []W	Birth Date: 7/21/52

Phone: 614-221-0202	SS#: 716-83-0061		

Address: 12 Briar Lane	Employer: Stephenson Wire Works		

City: Stephenson	State: OH	Zip: 60089	Employer's Address: 125 Stephenson Road

Student Status: full-time	City: Stephenson	State: OH	Zip: 60089

INSURANCE INFORMATION

Primary Insurance Company: Blue Cross Blue Shield	Secondary Insurance Company: Physician's Alliance of Ohio

Subscriber's Name: Juan Lomos	Birth Date: 7/21/52	Rel. to Insured: child	Subscriber's Name: Cedera Lomos	Birth Date: 5/21/57	Rel. to Insured: child

Plan: Traditional	SS#: 716-83-0061	Plan: Traditional	SS#: 717-87-0054

Policy #: 716830061	Group #: 126	Policy #: 621382	Group #: A435

Copayment/Deductible: $250 ded.	Price Code: A	Copayment/Deductible: $100 ded.	Price Code: A

OTHER INFORMATION

Reason for visit: Routine well-child checkup	Allergy to Medication (list):

Name of referring physician:	If auto accident, list date and state in which it occurred:

I authorize treatment and agree to pay all fees and charges for the person named above. I agree to pay all charges shown by statements, promptly upon their presentation, unless credit arrangements are agreed upon in writing.

I authorize payment directly to FAMILY MEDICAL GROUP of insurance benefits otherwise payable to me. I hereby authorize the release of any medical information necessary in order to process a claim for payment in my behalf.

Juan Lomos	9/3/10
(Patient's Signature/Parent or Guardian's Signature)	(Date)

I plan to make payment of my medical expenses as follows (check one or more):

<u>X</u> Insurance (as above)   <u>X</u> Cash/Check/Credit/Debit Card   _____ Medicare   _____ Medicaid   _____ Workers' Comp.

Figure 1-2   *Sample Patient Information Form*

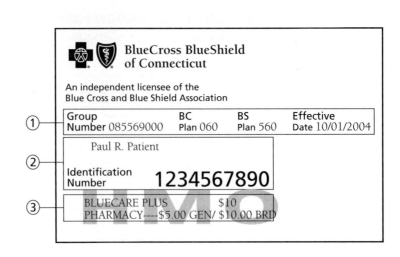

1. **Group identification number**
   The 9-digit number used to identify the member's employer.

   Blue Cross Blue Shield plan codes
   The numbers used to identify the codes assigned to each plan by the Blue Cross Blue Shield Association: used for claims submissions when medical services are rendered out-of-state.

   Effective date
   The date on which the member's coverage became effective.

2. **Member name**
   The full name of the cardholder.

   Identification number
   The 10-digit number used to identify each Anthem Blue Cross and Blue Shield of Connecticut or BlueCare Health Plan member.

3. **Health plan**
   The name of the health plan and the type of coverage; usually lists any copayment amounts, frequency limits or annual maximums for home and office visits; may also list the member's annual deductible amount.

   Riders
   The type(s) of riders that are included in the member's benefits (DME, Visions).

   Pharmacy
   The type of prescription drug coverage; lists copayment amounts.

Figure 1-3 *Sample Insurance Identification Card*

forms and statements. It is good practice to ask the patient to update information at every visit.

In addition to having a patient complete this form, the patient's insurance identification card is photocopied or scanned, and the patient's current eligibility and benefits are verified either online or over the phone (see Figure 1-3).

Table 1-1 shows the principal types of insurance carriers you will deal with.

In addition, you may deal with workers' compensation, a state-regulated type of insurance covering certain on-the-job injuries, or automobile insurance in the case of an auto accident.

Table 1-1	Types of Insurance Carriers
Carrier Description	**Description**
Blue Cross and Blue Shield	Nonprofit or for-profit plans with medical, surgical, and hospital benefits. Payments are often made directly to providers.
Commercial Insurers	Profit-making medical, surgical, and hospitalization insurance plans. Payments are often made directly to patients.
Medicare	Government health insurance for the elderly. Part A covers hospital services. Part B partially pays for doctor's services. Part D provides a prescription drug benefit. Payments are made to providers in most cases.
Medicaid (MediCal)	Government health insurance for low-income people. Payments are made to providers.
TRICARE and CHAMPVA	Government health insurance for dependents of certain military personnel (TRICARE) and for dependents of disabled veterans (CHAMPVA). Payments are made to providers.
Health Maintenance Organization (HMO)	A medical center or group of providers that provides medical services to patients for fixed monthly or annual fees. Payments are made to providers.
Preferred Provider Organization (PPO)	Insurer contracts with a group of providers who agree to provide care based on a predetermined list of charges. The providers bill the PPO directly.
Consumer-Driven Health Plan (CDHP)	Plan in which a high-deductible/low-premium insurance plan is combined with a pretax savings account to cover out-of-pocket medical expenses.

Step 4 Check Out Patients

Many medical offices use a case-based system to organize patient records. That is, all patient payments, insurance claim reimbursements, and adjustments are linked to a case. A **case** is a grouping of procedures or transactions generally organized by the type of treatment or insurance carrier. For every new case, a billing assistant must record the pertinent information, which includes the following: case description, guarantor, marital status, employer, provider, insurance carrier, policy number, and diagnosis. The **guarantor** is the person or party responsible for payment of a patient's medical bills.

On a daily basis, a billing assistant uses encounter forms to record case information, identify procedure charges, process patient payments, and make account adjustments. An **encounter form** (or superbill) is a document that lists all services performed for one patient in a single office visit. The form has places for the patient's name, medical services provided that day, diagnosis, amount of each individual charge for the day, total for the visit, and amount paid. A **diagnosis** is the doctor's determination of what is wrong with the patient, based on an examination.

A sample encounter form is shown in Figure 1-4. An encounter form is included in each patient's chart at the start of the visit. The doctor, laboratory technician, nurse, or anyone else who performs a procedure for the patient during that visit records the service on the encounter form. A **procedure** is a service performed, such as an office visit with a provider (including examination, evaluation of symptoms, and determination of a course of treatment), an injection, or a laboratory test. At the end of the visit, the assistant at the front desk uses the encounter form to calculate the total charge and to record any payment received. The form then goes to the medical billing assistant, who uses it to update the patient ledger and the day sheet.

To simplify the billing process, medical offices use a set of standard procedure codes known as **CPT-4** (*Current Procedural Terminology, Fourth Edition*). Procedures that are commonly performed in the practice are usually listed on the encounter form along with the corresponding CPT-4 code. For example, the sample encounter form shown in Figure 1-4 includes such procedure codes as 82951 (glucose tolerance test) and 85025 (CBC w/differential).These two codes would be marked if the patient had received a blood sugar tolerance test and a complete blood count.

As part of the patient case information, you must also record the diagnosis. A set of medical diagnosis codes known as **ICD-9-CM** (*International Classification of Diseases,* Ninth Revision, *Clinical Modification*) makes this task much easier. For instance, if a doctor wrote "diabetes mellitus" on a patient's encounter form, you would use the code for diabetes mellitus (250.00) to record the diagnosis. In the future, ICD-9-CM will be replaced with ICD-10-CM.

Every day as a billing assistant, you will record all payments received from patients and their insurance carriers. Patient payments may be made by cash, check, or credit card. When a payment is made, a receipt is given to the patient. In some medical offices, you may also be responsible for preparing a bank deposit slip. Each day, you will record all of the checks and cash received on a deposit slip and take the deposit to the bank. To verify that you recorded the day's receipts correctly, you can compare the bank deposit total with the day sheet total. The two totals should match.

ENCOUNTER FORM

7/9/10	11:30am
DATE	TIME

Dr. Katherine Yan	
PROVIDER	

Stanley Feldman	
PATIENT NAME	

FELST000	
CHART #	

OFFICE VISITS - SYMPTOMATIC - NEW		
99201	OF--New Patient Minimal	
99202	OF--New Patient Low	
99203	OF--New Patient Detailed	
99204	OF--New Patient Moderate	
99205	OF--New Patient High	
OFFICE VISITS - SYMPTOMATIC - ESTABLISHED		
99211	OF--Established Patient Minimal	
99212	OF--Established Patient Low	X
99213	OF--Established Patient Detailed	
99214	OF--Established Patient Moderate	
99215	OF--Established Patient High	
PREVENTIVE VISITS - NEW		
99381	Under 1 Year	
99382	1 - 4 Years	
99383	5 - 11 Years	
99384	12 - 17 Years	
99385	18 - 39 Years	
99386	40 - 64 Years	
99387	65 Years & Up	
PREVENTIVE VISITS - ESTABLISHED		
99391	Under 1 Year	
99392	1 - 4 Years	
99393	5 - 11 Years	
99394	12 - 17 Years	
99395	18 - 39 Years	
99396	40 - 64 Years	
99397	65 Years & Up	
PROCEDURES		
12011	Repair of superficial wounds, face	
29125	Short arm splint	
45378	Colonoscopy--diagnostic	
45380	Colonoscopy--biopsy	
71010	Chest x-ray, frontal	
71020	Chest x-ray, frontal and lateral	
73070	Elbow x-ray, AP and lateral	

PROCEDURES		
73090	Forearm x-ray, AP and lateral	
73100	Wrist x-ray, AP and lateral	
73600	Ankle x-ray, AP and lateral	
93000	Electrocardiogram--ECG	
93015	Treadmill stress test	
LABORATORY		
80061	Lipid panel	
82270	Hemoccult--stool screening	
82465	Cholesterol test	
82947	Glucose--quantitative	
82951	Glucose tolerance test	
83718	HDL cholesterol test	
85007	Manual WBC	
85025	CBC w/diff.	
85651	Erythrocyte sed rate--ESR	
86580	Mantoux test	
87040	Bacterial culture	
87430	Strep screen	
87086	Urine colony count	
87088	Urine culture	
INJECTIONS		
90465	Immunization administration, pt under 8 yrs	
90471	Immunization administration	
90657	Influenza injection, under 35 months	
90658	Influenza injection, older than 3 years	
90703	Tetanus immunization	
90707	MMR immunization	

PB FAMILY CARE CENTER

REFERRING PHYSICIAN	NPI

AUTHORIZATION #

DIAGNOSIS
848.9

PAYMENT AMOUNT
$10.00 copay, check #2944

NOTES

Figure 1-4   *Sample Encounter Form*

1. Which form is also referred to as a superbill?
2. What reference is used to find a procedure code?
3. What reference can be used to find a list of common diagnoses?

Step 5 Review Coding Compliance

The data on the encounter form must be checked for errors. Each procedure performed by a health care provider during an office visit is related to a specific diagnostic code. The diagnosis and the medical services received should be logically connected so that the medical necessity of the charges will be clear to the insurance company. The medical office staff member who does the coding must have specialized knowledge. In some medical practices, the physicians assign these codes; in others, a medical coder or a medical insurance specialist handles the task.

Step 6 Check Billing Compliance

Most medical practices have standard fee schedules listing their usual fees for procedures. The provider's fees for services are listed on the medical practice's fee schedule. However, the fees listed on the master fee schedule are not necessarily the amount the provider will be paid. Many providers enter into contracts with insurance plans that require discounts from standard fees. The billing program estimates the amount the provider will receive, based on the patient's insurance.

Step 7 Prepare and Transmit Claims

Very few patients pay all of their medical bills themselves. Most people have some kind of medical insurance to help cover the costs. A small number of patients file their own insurance claims; a patient who does so often attaches a copy of the encounter form to the claim form. For the most part, however, providers prepare health care claims for patients using billing software and then transmit the claims electronically to the patients' health plans.

It is the medical billing assistant's job to be sure that the claims are created and sent to insurance carriers. In addition to indicating the CPT-4 code and charges on the insurance claim, you will enter basic information about the patient and a code for the diagnosis. Most claims are transmitted electronically.

In the past, the paper **CMS-1500** form was the standard health claim accepted by most payers (see Figure 1-5). It was typed or computer-generated and mailed to payers. Sending paper claims became less common with the increased use of information technology (IT) in physician practices. HIPAA, with its emphasis on electronic transactions, has made the use of IT very common. HIPAA requires electronic transmission of claims, except by very small practices–those with less than ten full-time or equivalent employees and that never send any kind of electronic health care transactions. These excepted offices are the only providers that can still send paper claims. The electronic claim format for professional claims is known as the

HEALTH INSURANCE CLAIM FORM

APPROVED BY NATIONAL UNIFORM CLAIM COMMITTEE 08/05

☐☐ PICA

PICA ☐☐☐

CARRIER

1. MEDICARE MEDICAID TRICARE CHAMPUS CHAMPVA GROUP HEALTH PLAN FECA BLK LUNG OTHER	1a. INSURED'S I.D. NUMBER (For Program in Item 1)

☐ (Medicare #) ☐ (Medicaid #) ☐ (Sponsor's SSN) ☐ (Member ID#) ☐ (SSN or ID) ☐ (SSN) ☐ (ID)

2. PATIENT'S NAME (Last Name, First Name, Middle Initial)

3. PATIENT'S BIRTH DATE   MM | DD | YY   SEX   M ☐   F ☐

4. INSURED'S NAME (Last Name, First Name, Middle Initial)

5. PATIENT'S ADDRESS (No., Street)

6. PATIENT RELATIONSHIP TO INSURED   Self ☐ Spouse ☐ Child ☐ Other ☐

7. INSURED'S ADDRESS (No., Street)

CITY   STATE

8. PATIENT STATUS   Single ☐ Married ☐ Other ☐

CITY   STATE

ZIP CODE   TELEPHONE (Include Area Code)   (   )

Employed ☐   Full-Time Student ☐   Part-Time Student ☐

ZIP CODE   TELEPHONE (Include Area Code)   (   )

9. OTHER INSURED'S NAME (Last Name, First Name, Middle Initial)

10. IS PATIENT'S CONDITION RELATED TO:

11. INSURED'S POLICY GROUP OR FECA NUMBER

a. OTHER INSURED'S POLICY OR GROUP NUMBER

a. EMPLOYMENT? (Current or Previous)   ☐ YES ☐ NO

a. INSURED'S DATE OF BIRTH   MM | DD | YY   SEX   M ☐   F ☐

b. OTHER INSURED'S DATE OF BIRTH   MM | DD | YY   SEX   M ☐   F ☐

b. AUTO ACCIDENT?   PLACE (State)   ☐ YES ☐ NO

b. EMPLOYER'S NAME OR SCHOOL NAME

c. EMPLOYER'S NAME OR SCHOOL NAME

c. OTHER ACCIDENT?   ☐ YES ☐ NO

c. INSURANCE PLAN NAME OR PROGRAM NAME

d. INSURANCE PLAN NAME OR PROGRAM NAME

10d. RESERVED FOR LOCAL USE

d. IS THERE ANOTHER HEALTH BENEFIT PLAN?   ☐ YES ☐ NO   *If yes*, return to and complete item 9 a-d.

READ BACK OF FORM BEFORE COMPLETING & SIGNING THIS FORM.

12. PATIENT'S OR AUTHORIZED PERSON'S SIGNATURE I authorize the release of any medical or other information necessary to process this claim. I also request payment of government benefits either to myself or to the party who accepts assignment below.

SIGNED _____   DATE _____

13. INSURED'S OR AUTHORIZED PERSON'S SIGNATURE I authorize payment of medical benefits to the undersigned physician or supplier for services described below.

SIGNED _____

PATIENT AND INSURED INFORMATION

14. DATE OF CURRENT: MM | DD | YY   ◄ ILLNESS (First symptom) OR INJURY (Accident) OR PREGNANCY(LMP)

15. IF PATIENT HAS HAD SAME OR SIMILAR ILLNESS. GIVE FIRST DATE   MM | DD | YY

16. DATES PATIENT UNABLE TO WORK IN CURRENT OCCUPATION   MM | DD | YY   FROM   TO   MM | DD | YY

17. NAME OF REFERRING PROVIDER OR OTHER SOURCE

17a.

17b. NPI

18. HOSPITALIZATION DATES RELATED TO CURRENT SERVICES   MM | DD | YY   FROM   TO   MM | DD | YY

19. RESERVED FOR LOCAL USE

20. OUTSIDE LAB?   ☐ YES ☐ NO $ CHARGES

21. DIAGNOSIS OR NATURE OF ILLNESS OR INJURY (Relate Items 1, 2, 3 or 4 to Item 24E by Line)

1. └___ . ___┘   3. └___ . ___┘

2. └___ . ___┘   4. └___ . ___┘

22. MEDICAID RESUBMISSION CODE   ORIGINAL REF. NO.

23. PRIOR AUTHORIZATION NUMBER

24. A. DATE(S) OF SERVICE			B. PLACE OF SERVICE	C. EMG	D. PROCEDURES, SERVICES, OR SUPPLIES (Explain Unusual Circumstances)		E. DIAGNOSIS POINTER	F. $ CHARGES	G. DAYS OR UNITS	H. EPSDT Family Plan	I. ID. QUAL.	J. RENDERING PROVIDER ID. #
From MM DD YY	To MM DD YY				CPT/HCPCS	MODIFIER						
1											NPI	
2											NPI	
3											NPI	
4											NPI	
5											NPI	
6											NPI	

25. FEDERAL TAX I.D. NUMBER   SSN ☐ EIN ☐

26. PATIENT'S ACCOUNT NO.

27. ACCEPT ASSIGNMENT? (For govt. claims, see back)   ☐ YES ☐ NO

28. TOTAL CHARGE $

29. AMOUNT PAID $

30. BALANCE DUE

31. SIGNATURE OF PHYSICIAN OR SUPPLIER INCLUDING DEGREES OR CREDENTIALS (I certify that the statements on the reverse apply to this bill and are made a part thereof.)

SIGNED _____   DATE _____

32. SERVICE FACILITY LOCATION INFORMATION

a. NPI   b.

33. BILLING PROVIDER INFO & PH #   (   )

a. NPI   b.

PHYSICIAN OR SUPPLIER INFORMATION

NUCC Instruction Manual available at: www.nucc.org

Figure 1-5   *CMS-1500 Claim Form*

HIPAA x12N 837P, or 837P for short. The information on the HIPAA electronic transaction and the paper form, with a few exceptions, is the same.

Step 8 Monitor Payer Adjudication

When the claim is received by the payer, it is reviewed to determine whether it should be paid. Once accepted, claims may be paid in full, partially paid, or denied. The results of this process are explained in a document that is sent to the provider along with the payment. This document is called a remittance advice (RA) or explanation of benefits (EOB).

When a remittance advice is received from the insurance carrier, the billing assistant records payments. Depending on the rules of the health plan, the patient may be billed for an outstanding balance. In other circumstances, an account adjustment is made.

A new adjudication process known as **real-time claims adjudication (RTCA)** is increasingly used in computerized offices. With RTCA, a billing assistant submits claims at the time the patient checks out. Once a claim is submitted, assuming the payer has RTCA capabilities, the payor's computer system adjudicates the claim within minutes and sends back an EOB. The billing assistant then discusses the payer's decision with the patient in person, and the patient pays any balance due before leaving. If there is a problem with the claim, such as missing information, the billing assistant can work with the patient to resolve the problem and resubmit the claim. With most claims, there is no need to create a patient statement. The only follow up for the medical office is to verify that the payer's portion of the payment is received. Payment usually follows within twenty-four hours.

Step 9 Generate Patient Statements

Usually, a billing assistant prepares and mails patient statements once a month. The statements summarize the office visits and charges during the month, itemize payments on the accounts, and show the unpaid account balances. The statement is the patient's bill for services. In some practices, statements are sent on several days during each month. For example, patients whose last names begin with A to M may be billed on the fifteenth of the month and patients with last names beginning with N to Z may be billed on the last day of the month. Spreading out the billing means that there is less work to be done on a single day and that patient payments will be distributed more evenly throughout the month.

Step 10 Follow Up Payments and Collections

The **accounting cycle** is the flow of financial transactions in a business—from making a sale to collecting payment for the goods or services delivered. In a medical practice, this is the cycle from seeing and treating the patient to receiving payment for services provided. Practice management software can be used to track **accounts receivable (AR)**—monies that are coming into the practice—and to produce financial reports.

At the end of each day, a report is generated that lists all charges, payments, and adjustments entered during that day (see Figure 1-6). The day sheet is a list of patients, charges, and services performed each day. In a

Family Care Center
Patient Day Sheet
Ending 8/29/2011

Entry	Date	Document	POS	Description	Provider	Code	Modifier	Amount
BELHE000		**Herbert Bell**						
200	8/29/2011	1108290000	11		1	USLCOP		-15.00
199	8/29/2011	1108290000	11		1	93015		325.00
198	8/29/2011	1108290000	11		1	99212		44.00
		Patient's Charges $369.00		Patient's Receipts -$15.00	Adjustments $0.00		Patient Balance $708.00	
BRORA000		**Rachel Brown**						
201	8/29/2011	1108290000	11		1	99211		30.00
203	8/29/2011	1108290000	11		1	USLCOP		-15.00
202	8/29/2011	1108290000	11		1	83718		35.00
		Patient's Charges $65.00		Patient's Receipts -$15.00	Adjustments $0.00		Patient Balance $100.00	
FELST000		**Stanley Feldman**						
204	8/29/2011	1108290000	11		1	99212		44.00
205	8/29/2011	1108290000	11		1	93015		325.00
		Patient's Charges $369.00		Patient's Receipts $0.00	Adjustments $0.00		Patient Balance $694.00	
JOHMA000		**Marion Johnson**						
206	8/29/2011	1108290000	11		1	99215		135.00
209	8/29/2011	1108290000	11		1	BCBPAY		-228.00
208	8/29/2011	1108290000	11		1	71010		80.00
207	8/29/2011	1108290000	11		1	93000		70.00
		Patient's Charges $285.00		Patient's Receipts -$228.00	Adjustments $0.00		Patient Balance $363.00	
MITCA000		**Caroline Mitchell**						
210	8/29/2011	1108290000	11		1	99213		60.00
		Patient's Charges $60.00		Patient's Receipts $0.00	Adjustments $0.00		Patient Balance $120.00	
MITHE000		**Herbert Mitchell**						
211	8/29/2011	1108290000	11		1	99213		60.00
		Patient's Charges $60.00		Patient's Receipts $0.00	Adjustments $0.00		Patient Balance $120.00	
PETAN000		**Ann Peterson**						
213	8/29/2011	1108290000	11		1	TRICOP		-10.00
212	8/29/2011	1108290000	11		1	99201		55.00
		Patient's Charges $55.00		Patient's Receipts -$10.00	Adjustments $0.00		Patient Balance $90.00	

Figure 1-6 *Sample Patient Day Sheet*

(continued)

manual system, a billing assistant must prepare the day sheet from the individual encounter forms and case reports. Day sheets have columns with headings such as Entry, Date, Document, Description, Provider, Code, and Amount. New charges, payments, and adjustments and the current balance are shown for each patient. A summary of the day's activity appears at the end of the report. To balance out a day, transactions listed on

```
                Family Care Center
        Patient Day Sheet
               Ending 8/29/2011

                    Total # Patients                            7
                    Total # Procedures                          12
                    Total Procedure Charges            $1,263.00
                    Total Product Charges                  $0.00
                    Total Inside Lab Charges               $0.00
                    Total Outside Lab Charges              $0.00
                    Total Billing Charges                  $0.00
                    Total Tax Charges                      $0.00
                    Total Charges                      $1,263.00

                    Total Insurance Payments            -$228.00
                    Total Cash Copayments                  $0.00
                    Total Check Copayments               -$40.00
                    Total Credit Card Copayments           $0.00
                    Total Patient Cash Payments            $0.00
                    Total Patient Check Payments           $0.00
                    Total Credit Card Payments             $0.00
                    Total Receipts                      -$268.00

                    Total Credit Adjustments               $0.00
                    Total Debit Adjustments                $0.00
                    Total Insurance Debit Adjustments      $0.00
                    Total Insurance Credit Adjustments     $0.00
                    Total Insurance Withholds              $0.00
                    Total Adjustments                      $0.00
                    Net Effect on Accounts Receivable    $995.00

            Practice Totals
                    Total # Procedures                     49
                    Total Charges                     $4,530.60
                    Total Payments                    -$512.60
                    Total Adjustments                      $0.00

                    Accounts Receivable               $4,018.00
```

Figure 1-6   *Sample Patient Day Sheet (continued)*

encounter forms (charges and payments) and totals from bank deposit entries are compared against the end-of-day report. Day sheets are also used to balance accounts at the end of every month.

A monthly report summarizes the financial activity of the entire month. This report lists charges, payments, and adjustments and the total accounts receivable for the month. It is possible to balance out the month by totaling the daily charges, payments, and adjustments and then comparing the totals to the amounts listed on the monthly report.

It is also good practice to frequently print reports that list the outstanding balances owed to the practice by health plans or patients. Regular review of these reports can alert the billing staff to accounts that require action to collect the amount due. A sample **patient ledger** is illustrated in Figure 1-7. The patient ledger report includes the patient's name, procedure date and code, provider, charges, payments, adjustments, and account balance.

Family Care Center
Patient Account Ledger
From August 1, 2011 to August 31, 2011

Entry	Date	POS	Description	Procedure	Document	Provider	Amount
BELHE000		**Herbert Bell**		(614)241-6124			
		Last Payment: -15.00	On: 8/29/2011				
200	8/29/2011			USLCOP	1108290000	1	-15.00
199	8/29/2011			93015	1108290000	1	325.00
198	8/29/2011			99212	1108290000	1	44.00
		Patient Totals					354.00
BRORA000		**Rachel Brown**		(614)721-0044			
		Last Payment: -15.00	On: 8/29/2011				
201	8/29/2011			99211	1108290000	1	30.00
203	8/29/2011			USLCOP	1108290000	1	-15.00
202	8/29/2011			83718	1108290000	1	35.00
		Patient Totals					50.00
FELST000		**Stanley Feldman**		(614)555-9295			
		Last Payment: 0.00	On:				
204	8/29/2011			99212	1108290000	1	44.00
205	8/29/2011			93015	1108290000	1	325.00
		Patient Totals					369.00
JOHMA000		**Marion Johnson**		(614)726-9898			
		Last Payment: -228.00	On: 8/29/2011				
206	8/29/2011			99215	1108290000	1	135.00
209	8/29/2011			BCBPAY	1108290000	1	-228.00
208	8/29/2011			71010	1108290000	1	80.00
207	8/29/2011			93000	1108290000	1	70.00
		Patient Totals					57.00
MITCA000		**Caroline Mitchell**		(614)861-0909			
		Last Payment: 0.00	On:				
210	8/29/2011			99213	1108290000	1	60.00
		Patient Totals					60.00
MITHE000		**Herbert Mitchell**		(614)861-0909			
		Last Payment: 0.00	On:				
211	8/29/2011			99213	1108290000	1	60.00
		Patient Totals					60.00
PETAN000		**Ann Peterson**		(614)555-8989			
		Last Payment: -10.00	On: 8/29/2011				
213	8/29/2011			TRICOP	1108290000	1	-10.00
212	8/29/2011			99201	1108290000	1	55.00
		Patient Totals					45.00

Figure 1-7 *Sample Patient Ledger*

(continued)

Family Care Center
Patient Account Ledger
From August 1, 2011 to August 31, 2011

Entry	Date	POS	Description	Procedure	Document	Provider	Amount
	Ledger Totals						995.00
	Accounts Receivable Total						$4,018.00

Figure 1-7   *Sample Patient Ledger (continued)*

The patient ledger lists all the activity for each patient account. To complete this ledger, a billing assistant enters the required information from the encounter form and day sheet. Since some patients do not pay when services are provided, it is very important for the office to keep a record of how much each patient owes. The patient ledger report serves as an internal record that shows the amount each patient owes. A collection process is often started when patient payments are later than permitted under the practice's financial policy.

✓CHECKPOINT

4. Which ledger is used to track all the activity for a patient?

5. Which report shows the patients seen, charges recorded, and services performed each day?

6. If paper insurance claims are filed, what is the name of the form that is typically used?

Computerized Medical Office Databases

As you have learned, the major documents used or produced in a patient billing system are encounter forms, day sheets, patient ledgers, patient statements, insurance forms, and patient information forms. Important information is recorded on each of these documents, and information from one document is often used in the preparation of others.

In a typical medical office using a manual system, basic information about each patient's visit is

1. Recorded first on an encounter form.

2. Transferred from an encounter form to a day sheet.

3. Posted from an encounter form or day sheet to the patient ledger.

4. Used in preparing an insurance form for the visit.

5. Included on the patient statement for the month.

All information collected and recorded on the various documents in an office can be considered part of a medical office database. A **database** is a collection of information (data) arranged logically so that it can be stored and retrieved. In a medical office where all records are kept manually, the database consists of paper records kept in files.

When a computerized patient billing system is used, the database is maintained by the computer. Backup copies of data are filed in the office or in a secure offsite location so that they can be retrieved in the event of computer problems.

A computerized medical billing program, such as Medisoft, stores these major types of data:

- **Provider Data**   The provider database has information about the physician(s) as well as the practice, such as its name and address, telephone number, and tax and medical identifier numbers.

- **Patient Data**   Information on each patient is stored in the patient database. The patient's unique chart number and personal information—name and address, telephone number, birth date, Social Security number, gender, marital status, and employer—are examples of information stored in this database.

- **Insurance Carriers**   The insurance carrier database contains the names, addresses, and other data about each insurance carrier used by patients, such as the type of plan. Usually, this database also contains information on each carrier's electronic claim submission.

- **Diagnosis Codes**   The diagnosis code database contains the ICD-9-CM codes that indicate the reason a service is provided. The codes entered in this database are those most frequently used by the practice.

- **Procedure Codes**   The procedure code database contains the data needed to create charges. The CPT-4 codes most often used by the practice are selected for this database. Other claim data elements, such as place of service (POS) and the charge for each procedure, are also stored in the procedure code database.

- **Transactions**   The transaction database stores information about each patient's visits, diagnoses, and procedures as well as about received and outstanding payments. **Transactions** in the form of charges, payments, and adjustments are also stored in the transaction database.

Within Medisoft, each database is linked, or related, to each of the others by having at least one fact in common. For example, information entered in the patient database is shared with the transaction database, linking the two. Information is entered only once; Medisoft selects the data from each database as needed.

Information stored in a medical office database is used for a variety of purposes. For example, the patient **data file** is used to update patient ledgers, create patient statements, and prepare insurance claims. When you work with a computerized patient billing system, you may not be aware of how much of the database is being used. The computerized system allows you to automatically retrieve data from and add new data to the database as you work.

Comparing a Computerized Billing System with a Manual Billing System

As you have learned in this chapter, the Medisoft program includes numerous options that can be used by a medical billing assistant to maintain a computerized patient accounting system. A patient accounting program such as Medisoft offers many advantages over a manual system. Several advantages of a computerized system are discussed in the following sections.

Access to Information

With a computer database, all the information is located in one place. Pieces of paper and forms are not located in different file cabinets in the office; they are all stored on one computer system.

In addition, computer data can be used by more than one person at a time. If an office has more than one computer, the computers can be linked together in a network, which allows them to share files in the central database. In an office without a computer database, it is difficult for someone to update a document if another person is working on it.

HIPAA Tip > The **HIPAA Security Rule** outlines the required administrative, technical, and physical safeguards to prevent unauthorized access to protected health care information. The security standards help safeguard confidential health information.

As one security measure, many medical offices assign passwords to individuals who have access to computer files, thereby limiting access to data stored on the computer. Access is granted on an as-needed basis. For example, the individual responsible for scheduling may not be able to access medical records or billing data. On the other hand, the physicians and several others (such as the practice manager) most likely have access to all databases.

As additional security, computer programs keep track of data entry and create an audit trail—a way to trace who has accessed information and when. When new information is entered or existing data are changed, a log is created to record the time and date of the entry as well as the name of the computer operator. This log is stored and may be reviewed by the practice manager on a regular basis to detect irregularities. In addition, the program lists the name of the operator and the date information was entered, making it possible to identify an operator if an error has been made.

Search Capability

Another advantage of computer databases is the simplicity of conducting a search for information. Instead of having to look in different file cabinets and folders, a search can be conducted by entering a few keystrokes. In a very short time, the information is retrieved and displayed on the computer screen.

Minimal Storage Space

Computers also eliminate the need for large amounts of physical storage space, since much of the information is stored in the computer and not on paper.

Prod

Bringing computers into the medical office has greatly increased productivity, primarily because computers are much more efficient at processing large amounts of data than are human beings. Tasks that would take minutes for a person to complete can be done by the computer in a matter of seconds. For example, suppose a medical practice has multiple providers and hundreds of patients. A patient calls to ask about the amount owed on an account. With a computerized billing program in place, the medical office assistant might simply key the first few letters of the patient's last name into the computer, causing the patient's account to appear on the screen. The outstanding balance could then be communicated to the patient.

In another example, suppose the wrong diagnosis code has been written on an insurance claim form and the claim has been rejected by the insurance carrier. To resubmit the claim without the use of a computer might require completing the entire form again by hand. However, if the medical office used a computerized billing program, the error could be corrected in seconds and a new claim submitted electronically.

Electronic Claims Transmission

An electronic claim is an insurance claim that is sent electronically from one computer to another, using a phone line, cable line, or via satellite. Today, most insurance claims are transmitted electronically using the standard electronic format, the 837P, mandated by HIPAA. Electronic claim filing has several advantages. First, it is faster to file and process claims electronically than to fill out and process paper forms, and doing so requires fewer staff members. In addition, it costs less to file electronically; the costs of paper forms, envelopes, and postage are much higher than the costs of electronic transmission.

Fewer Errors

Computers not only make the medical office more efficient, but also reduce the number of errors. Working with a computer system, information is entered once and used over and over again. Provided the information is entered correctly the first time, it will be correct every time it is used. For example, information such as the patient's address and insurance policy number is entered in the computer once. The computer stores the information, locates it when it is time to create a claim, and uses it to complete the task. The next time a claim needs to be created, the computer goes through the same process, using the same information. Without a computer, someone would have to key all the information on an insurance form each time a claim was being submitted for the patient. Not only does this consume more time, but it also introduces the possibility of error every time the information is rekeyed.

While computers do increase the efficiency of the medical office and reduce the number of errors, they are not more accurate than the individual entering the data. If human errors occur while entering information, the data coming out of the computer will be incorrect. Computers are very precise and also very unforgiving. While the human brain knows that *flu* is short for *influenza*, the computer does not know this, and it regards them as two distinct conditions. If a computer operator accidentally enters a name as ORourke instead of O'Rourke, a person might know what is meant; the computer does not. It would probably respond to a request for the ORourke file with a message such as "No such patient exists in the database."

Most human errors occur during data entry, such as pressing the wrong key on the keyboard, or because of the lack of computer literacy—not knowing how to use a program to accomplish the tasks. For this reason, proper training in the use of computer programs is essential for medical office personnel.

Claims Creation and Processing

From an administrative perspective, the most significant use of the computer in the medical office is to create and process insurance claims. When preparing patients' claims, the computer selects information from its databases to create an electronic claim file, which is transmitted electronically.

Fewer Steps to Record Data

One important advantage is that a computerized system eliminates unnecessary steps. For example, Medisoft allows you to enter data in one place and then automatically uses that information in many other areas. Once data has been entered into the system, creating any number of reports is as simple as clicking the mouse.

Table 1-2 identifies the steps to transfer information from the encounter form to prepare a day sheet and a patient ledger. The steps in a manual system are compared with the steps in a computerized system. As you can see, many of the steps required in a manual system are performed automatically by a patient accounting program such as Medisoft.

Table 1-2 Manual System versus Computerized System

Manual System	Computerized System
Provider fills out an encounter form, and a person at the front desk totals the charge and collects payment.	Same.
Medical billing assistant writes the encounter form information on a day sheet.	Medical billing assistant enters the procedure and diagnosis information in the computer.
Medical billing assistant totals columns on a day sheet at the end of a day.	Totals for the day are automatically updated by the program.
Medical billing assistant uses a day sheet at the end of a day to write information on the patient ledgers.	Patient ledgers are automatically updated by the program.
Medical billing assistant calculates each patient's new balance.	New balances are automatically calculated by the program.

Chapter 1 Review

Define the Terms

Write a definition for each term: (Obj. 1-1)

1. Case

   _____

2. Consumer-driven health plan

   _____

3. CPT-4

   _____

4. Day sheet

   _____

5. Encounter form

   _____

6. Guarantor

   _____

7. HIPAA Security Rule

   _____

8. ICD-9-CM

   _____

9. Patient ledger

   _____

10. Procedure

    _____

11. Transactions

    _____

12. List five important financial records that are kept by a medical office. (Objs. 1-2 and 1-4)

_____

_____

_____

_____

_____

13. List four types of government health plans, along with the population group they represent. (Obj. 1-3)

_____

_____

_____

_____

14. Who in the medical office fills out the encounter form? Who uses the information on the encounter form and for what purposes? (Obj. 1-3)

_____

_____

_____

_____

15. What are the ten steps in the medical billing process? (Obj. 1-3)

_____

_____

_____

_____

16. Similar information is found on a day sheet and a patient ledger. What is the difference between these two forms? (Obj. 1-4)

_____

_____

_____

_____

17. What is the principal responsibility of the medical billing assistant? (Objs. 1-3 and 1-4)

_____

_____

_____

_____

18. List and describe the six major types of data that are part of the Medisoft database. (Obj. 1-5)

_____

_____

_____

_____

19. Describe the advantages of a computerized billing system over a manual patient accounting system. (Obj. 1-6)

_____

_____

_____

_____

CRITICAL ANALYSIS EXERCISE

20. From a financial point of view, what is the role and importance of patient billing in the medical office? (Obj. 1-2)

_____

_____

_____

Using the Computer for Patient Billing

WHAT YOU NEED TO KNOW

To complete this chapter, you need to know:

- What the major elements of a medical office accounting system are and how patient billing fits into the system.
- The main responsibilities of a medical billing assistant.
- What financial records the medical billing assistant maintains and what each record contains.

WHAT YOU WILL LEARN

When you finish this chapter, you will be able to complete the following objectives:

2-1. Define the terms used in this chapter.

2-2. Define the options available in a computerized patient accounting system.

2-3. Start and exit Medisoft.

2-4. Make selections from Medisoft menus.

2-5. Explain the importance of dates in Medisoft.

KEY TERMS

Knowledge base Searchable collection of updated information about a topic.

Medisoft Program Date The date used by the Medisoft program to process transactions. Unless specifically set, the program uses the current date stored by the computer.

Menu bar Listing of menus, from which options are selected, within a program.

Toolbar A bar located below the menu bar that provides an alternate method of accessing program options. Icons provide rapid access to program options.

Medisoft: A Computerized Patient Billing System

A computerized patient billing system allows you to perform many, if not all, of the tasks performed in a manual system. The menus and submenus in the Medisoft system provide access to the program features needed to maintain a patient accounting system.

Medisoft Menu Bar

The Medisoft main window, shown in Figure 2-1, appears after you start the program. The **menu bar** is the main menu that appears horizontally across the top of an application's window. It lists the names of the menus in Medisoft: File, Edit, Activities, Lists, Reports, Tools, Window, Services, and Help. Beneath each menu name is a pull-down menu of one or more options. The options shown in the menu bar represent the categories of features available in the Medisoft program. As a medical billing assistant, most likely you will not use all these options; some are used by other staff members. The information in Table 2-1 describes most of the options available in the Medisoft program and explains which options a medical billing assistant would use.

As presented in Table 2-1, the Medisoft program organizes the program options by category. For example, all the reports are grouped in the Reports menu. To print the Patient Day Sheet report, you would pull down the Reports menu, choose the Day Sheets option, and then choose Patient Day Sheet. Figure 2-2 on page 33 shows the options in the Reports menu.

Figure 2-1   *Medisoft Main Window with Menu Bar*

Table 2-1 Medisoft Menu and Options

Menu	Options	Description	Used in Billing
FILE			
	Open Practice	Allows you to open a database file for a medical practice. This option is useful if you are using Medisoft for more than one practice.	Only indirectly to open a practice database.
	New Practice	Creates a new database for a medical practice.	No; usually others will set up a practice.
	Convert Data	Allows you to convert data from earlier versions of Medisoft.	No.
	Backup Data	Allows you to back up data.	Yes; for making a backup of a medical practice's database.
	Task Scheduler	Allows you to schedule tasks at a specified time.	Yes; for performing tasks during less busy times of the day.
	View Backup Disks	Lets you view data on a backup disk.	Yes.
	Restore Data	Restores data from a backup disk.	Yes.
	Backup Root Data	Creates a backup copy of root data.	Yes.
	Restore Root Data	Restores root data.	Yes.
	Set Program Date	Changes the date used by Medisoft to process data.	Yes.
	Practice Information	Allows you to make changes in an existing practice.	No.
	Program Options	Set backup parameters, startup options, and data-entry conventions.	No; most program options will already be configured.
	Security Setup	Set up features to ensure the security of the database.	No; will already be configured.
	Login/Password Management	Permits changes to allowed logins and passwords.	No; will be configured by office manager.
	Global Login Management	A security feature that sets up a path to enable a single user to access multiple practices without having to log in to each data set separately.	No; if required, will already be configured.
	File Maintenance	Lets you rebuild a medical office database and perform other maintenance options.	Yes; but only if the database files are damaged or need to be purged.
	Exit	Quits the program.	Yes.

(continued)

| Table 2-1 | Medisoft Menu and Options (continued) |

Menu	Options	Description	Used in Billing
EDIT			
	Cut Copy Paste Delete	All these options provide editing capabilities while you input data. You can use the cut, copy, and paste options to make processing data more efficient.	Yes; while entering data into the system.
ACTIVITIES			
	Enter Transactions	Allows you to record payments and deposits from patients and insurance carriers.	Yes.
	Claim Management	Provides options to create and print claim forms or send them electronically.	Yes.
	Statement Management	Allows you to create and print patient statements.	Yes.
	Enter Deposits/Payments	Allows you to record payments and deposits from patients and insurance carriers.	Yes.
	Unprocessed Transactions	Provides controls to both edit and post financial transactions imported from an electronic medical records (EMR) service.	Yes; if the practice subscribes to an EMR service.
	Patient Ledger	Displays the ledger of the selected patient.	Yes.
	Guarantor Ledger	Displays the ledger of the selected guarantor.	Yes.
	Quick Balance	Displays a summary of a patient's balance.	Yes.
	Patient Quick Entry	Lets you set up templates for the quick entry of patient data.	May already be configured by office manager.
	Billing Charges	Provides option to add billing charges to a patient's account.	Yes; if the practice uses billing charges.
	Small Balance Write-off	Writes off balances of less than a specified dollar amount.	Will already be configured by office manager.
	Collection List Add Collection List Item	Helps you manage financial transactions that need to be singled out for collections.	Yes.

Table 2-1   Medisoft Menu and Options (continued)

Menu	Options	Description	Used in Billing
ACTIVITIES			
	Launch Work Administrator	Launches the Work Administrator program, which functions like a to-do list.	Yes.
	Final Draft	A word-processing program that can be used to enter patient notes, letters, or other documents.	Yes; if the practice uses this feature.
	Add New Task	Used to add a work task to the Assignment List inside the Work Administrator program.	No; new tasks will be added by the practice manager.
	Appointment Book	Can be used to schedule patient appointments, repeating appointments, or other activities for each provider.	No; other staff members are usually responsible for scheduling.
	Eligibility Verification	Allows a patient's insurance eligibility status to be checked online.	Yes.
	Claims Manager	An add-on program that enables you to send electronic claims to a clearinghouse or directly to a payer; also performs claim edits and allows you to fix and resend claims and download response and remittance files.	Yes; if the practice has subscribed to the service.
LISTS			
	Patients/Guarantors and Cases Patient Recall Patient Treatment Plans Patient Para Template Procedure/Payment/ Adjustment Codes MultiLink Codes Diagnosis Codes Insurance Addresses EDI Receivers Referring Providers Provider Billing Codes Contact List Claim Rejection Messages Patient Payment Plan	The options in the Lists menu allow you to update all the data files or lists stored in a medical office's database. For example, you would use the Patients/Guarantors and Cases option to add new patient information or to update an existing patient's information.	Yes.

(continued)

| Table 2-1 | Medisoft Menu and Options (continued) |

Menu	Options	Description	Used in Billing
REPORTS	Day Sheets Analysis Reports Aging Reports Collection Reports Audit Reports Patient Ledger Standard Patient Lists Patient Statements Electronic Statements Claims Manager Reports Superbills Custom Report List Load Saved Reports Design Custom Reports and Bills	Provides access to reports, including patient ledgers, day sheets, and procedure day sheets. You can also create your own custom reports and bills.	Yes.
TOOLS	Calculator Medisoft Terminal View File Add/Copy User Reports Design Custom Patient Data Advanced Reporting AR2 Bundle Importer Communication Manager Administrative Dashboard Statement Wizard Collection Letter Wizard Electronic Remittance Customize Menu Bars System Information Modem Check User Information Patient Notes Patient Narrative	Provides access to tools, such as a calculator, a utility to view the content of a file, and an option to examine information about your computer.	No; except for the calculator if you need to manually calculate a charge. Most of the options would be used by other staff members, such as the program manager.
WINDOW	Close All Windows Minimize All Windows Tile Windows Horizontally Tile Windows Vertically Show Sidebar Clear Windows Positions Clear Custom Grid Settings Clear Saved Message Box Selections	Allows you to switch between windows (e.g., Patient List and Diagnosis List) used by the program.	Not directly; these options are used to change the window layout; they do not affect billing.

Table 2-1   Medisoft Menu and Options (continued)

Menu	Options	Description	Used in Billing
SERVICES	Claims Manager Eligibility Verification Electronic Prescribing Check for Update	The options on the Services menu are used to subscribe to add-on programs, such as Claims Manager, that can be used with Medisoft and to check for updates to Medisoft program files.	No; enrollment will be handled by office manager.
HELP	Medisoft Help Getting Started Upgraders from Medisoft for DOS Medisoft on the Web Online Updates Show Hints Show Shortcut Keys Register Program About Medisoft	Provides detailed information about each of Medisoft's options. Also includes information needed to register the program and to identify which version of the Medisoft program is being used.	Not directly; the options in this menu provide information to help you use the program more efficiently.

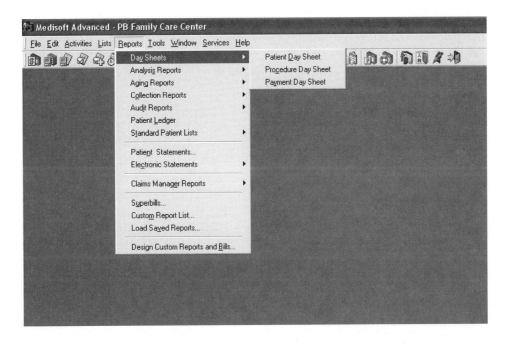

Figure 2-2   *Medisoft Window with Reports Menu Displayed*

Figure 2-3   *Medisoft Toolbar*

Toolbar

The **toolbar,** located just below the menu bar, provides icons for quick access to commonly used program functions (Figure 2-3). Many of the options in the Activities menu can be selected from the toolbar. Also, many of the Lists menu options, as well as the Custom Report List option from the Reports menu and the Medisoft Help option from the Help menu, can be selected by clicking the corresponding button on the toolbar.

√CHECKPOINT

1. A new patient visits the office and is treated for allergies. Which option from the Lists menu would you use to enter the patient and case information?

2. You need to print a day sheet at the end of a day. Which option would you choose to print this report?

3. What is the purpose of the Medisoft toolbar?

Getting Started with Medisoft

Before a medical office begins to use Medisoft, basic information about the practice and its patients must be entered in the program. This preliminary work has been done for you. The medical practice with which you will work is called PB Family Care Center. Check with your instructor to determine whether the Medisoft Student Data files (which contain the PB Family Care Center database) have already been loaded on your computer.

If your instructor has not already loaded the files, go to the Online Learning Center at www.mhhe.com/patientbilling7e to download them at this time. You will need to load the Medisoft Student Data files before you do the exercises in this chapter.

Navigating the Medisoft Menus

Once the Medisoft Student Data files are installed, you are ready to begin working with the Medisoft program. If you are familiar with other Microsoft Windows applications, you should be comfortable using the Medisoft program. Follow the steps in Computer Practice 2-1 to practice choosing options from the menu bar (see Figure 2-4).

Figure 2-4 *Medisoft Menu Bar*

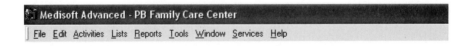

Computer Practice 2-1: *Using the Medisoft Menu Bar*

Follow these steps to choose an option from the Medisoft menu.

1. Position the mouse pointer on the Lists menu, and press the left mouse button once to display the menu options.

2. Move the mouse pointer to highlight the Diagnosis Codes option, and click the mouse button again to select the option.

3. The Diagnosis List window should appear on your screen. Using the options available in this window, you could add, edit, or delete diagnosis codes for the medical practice.

4. Click the Close button shown at the bottom of the Diagnosis List window to close the window.

5. Position the mouse pointer on the Diagnosis Code List button in the toolbar, and click the mouse button. As you can see, the toolbar provides another method of selecting an option from a Medisoft menu.

6. Close the Diagnosis List window.

7. Click each of the Medisoft menus to view the available options.

Dates

$ BILLING TIP

Instead of choosing the Set Program Date option, you can simply click the program date on the status bar in the lower right corner of the window to access this option.

Medisoft is a date-sensitive program. When transactions are entered in the program, if the dates are not accurate, the data entered will be of little value to the practice. Many times, date-sensitive information is not entered into Medisoft on the same day that the event or transaction occurred. For example, Friday afternoon's office visits may not be entered into the program until Monday. If the **Medisoft Program Date** is not changed to Friday's date before entering the data, all the information entered on Monday will be stored as Monday's transactions. For this reason, it is important to know how to change the Medisoft Program Date.

Changing the Medisoft Program Date

For most of the exercises in this book, you will need to change the Medisoft Program Date to the date specified at the beginning of the exercise. When the Medisoft program is started, the Medisoft Program Date is set to the computer's system date. The following steps are used to change the Medisoft Program Date:

1. Click Set Program Date on the File menu, or click the date displayed on the status bar. A pop-up calendar is displayed with the current date (see Figure 2-5).

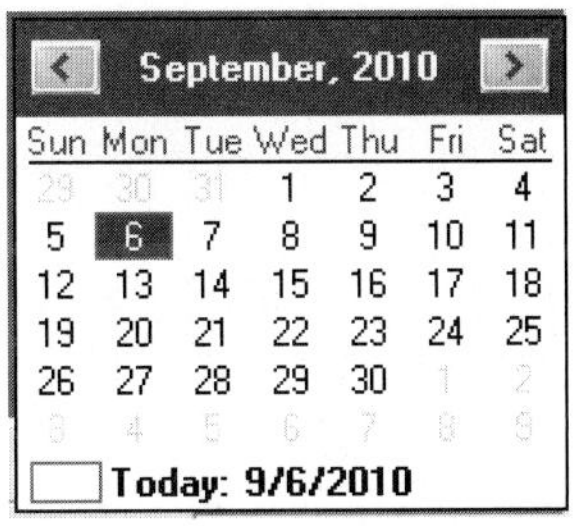

Figure 2-5   *Pop-up Calendar*

$ BILLING TIP

On computers using Vista, when the month is clicked on the pop-up calendar, the calendar window itself switches temporarily to a table of months rather than displaying a submenu of months. Select the desired month by clicking it in the table. Then, to select the year, first click the current year displayed on the table of months. A table of years, similar to the table of months, is displayed, with the decade listed above it. Click the desired year.

2. To change the date, click the name of the month that is currently displayed. A pop-up submenu with a list of months appears. Click the desired month.

3. Select the desired year by clicking the year that is currently displayed. A pop-up submenu listing two columns of years, up to the year 2009, appears. Click the desired year. *Note:* On computers using the Windows

BILLING TIP

On the pop-up calendar, the date displayed at the bottom of the calendar, labeled "Today," is the Windows or Vista System Date—the current date on the computer you are using. Do not click this date. If you do, the pop-up calendar will change to automatically display your computer's system date.

XP or earlier versions of Medisoft, for years after 2009, you must select 2009 and then use the right arrow button in the calendar window to advance one month at a time until you reach the desired year. With the Vista version, this step is not necessary; the calendar window itself switches to a table of years that includes the year 2010 and beyond.

4. Select the desired day of the month by clicking that date in the calendar.

5. If the date, month, or year you have selected is in the future, a pop-up message appears after you finish setting the day of the month to remind you that you have selected a future date (see Figure 2-6). To continue with the date change, click the OK button. (*Note*: Because the case studies for the exercises in this text/workbook take place in the year 2010, you may see this message often. Variations of the same message appear when entering future dates for patient visit transactions and deposits. Carefully read the message that is displayed; depending on the context, click Yes, No, or OK to continue with the date change.)

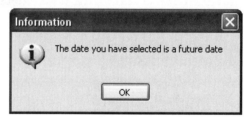

Figure 2-6   *Information Dialog Box That Appears When a Future Date Is Entered*

6. After setting the day of the month on the pop-up calendar, the calendar closes and the desired date is displayed on the status bar.

Formats for Entering Dates

In most Medisoft dialog boxes, dates can be entered in one of two formats, the MMDDCCYY format or the M/D/Y format. The MMDDCCYY format is a specific way in which dates are keyed. *MM* stands for the month, *DD* stands for the day, *CC* represents century, and *YY* stands for the year. Each day, month, century, and year entry must contain two digits, and no punctuation can be used. When dates are entered in this format, the program automatically adds slashes for you. For example, February 1, 2010, is keyed "02012010" and is displayed on the screen as "2/1/2010."

The other way of entering dates is to key the slashes manually. Using this method, you do not need to use double digits—the slashes indicate the divisions between month, day, and year. For example, you would key "2/1/10" or "2/1/2010" to enter February 1, 2010. Medisoft accepts either format for entering dates. As an alternative to keying dates, in many fields a pop-up calendar is available for entering a date.

Using Medisoft Help

Medisoft offers users three different types of help.

Hints   When the cursor moves over certain fields, text that explains the purpose of the field appears on the status bar at the bottom of the screen (see Figure 2-7).

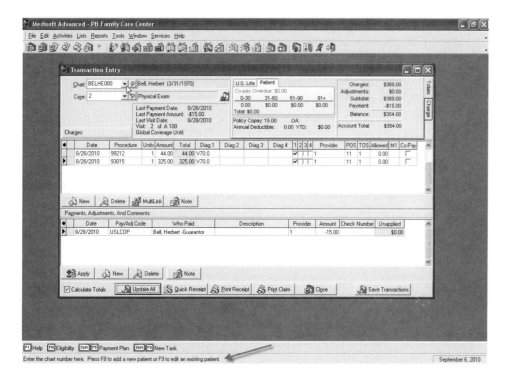

Figure 2-7 *Hints Help Feature*

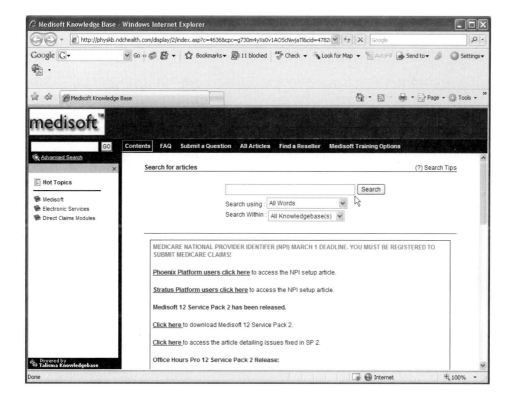

Figure 2-8 *Medisoft Online Knowledge Base*

Built-in Help   For more detailed help, Medisoft has an extensive help feature built into the program itself that is accessed through the Help menu.

Online Help   The Help menu also provides access to Medisoft help available on the Medisoft corporate website at www.Medisoft.com. The website contains a searchable **knowledge base,** which is a collection of up-to-date technical information about all Medisoft products (see Figure 2-8).

Computer Practice 2-2: *Using Medisoft's Built-in Help*

Follow the steps below to use the built-in help feature:

1. Click the Help menu and select Medisoft Help, or press function key F1.

2. On the left side of the Help window, click the Index tab.

3. Medisoft displays a list of topics for which help is available.

4. Click inside the text box at the top of the list to activate it, and then key *Diagnosis Entry* to locate this topic in the list. Double click on the highlighted topic name.

5. Information on entering diagnosis codes is displayed on the right side of the Help window.

6. Print the information by clicking the Print button at the top of the Help window. The Print dialog box is displayed.

7. Click the Print button to print.

8. To exit Help, click the X button in the top right corner of the Help window. You are returned to the main Medisoft window.

Computer Practice 2-3: *Using Medisoft's Online Help*

Go to Medisoft's website, and explore the knowledge base.

1. Select Medisoft on the Web on the Help menu, and then select Knowledge Base from the submenu.

2. Key the word *diagnosis* in the Search box, and review the knowledge base entries.

3. Close the website Help window by clicking the X button in the top right corner of the window. You are returned to the main Medisoft window.

Exiting Medisoft

When you finish using the Medisoft program at the end of each class or lab, you need to back up your data and exit the program. Since you have not made any changes to the database in this chapter, you do not need to make a backup this time. Backing up data is covered in the next chapter.

There are three ways to exit the Medisoft program:

1. Click Exit on the File menu.

2. Click the Exit button (the rightmost button) on the Medisoft toolbar.

3. Click the X button in the top right corner of the window.

TAKE NOTE: If your data are on a removable storage device, do not remove the device until you completely exit the Medisoft program.

✓CHECKPOINT

4. What are the three types of Help available in Medisoft?

5. By default, Medisoft uses the computer's operating system date as the Medisoft Program Date. How do you change the Medisoft Program Date to something other than the system date?

6. What menu would you use to add a new diagnosis code to Medisoft?

Chapter 2 Review

Define the Terms

Write a definition for each term: (Obj. 2-1)

1. Knowledge base

   _____

2. Medisoft Program Date

   _____

3. Menu bar

   _____

4. Toolbar

   _____

Check Your Understanding

5. What are the menus listed on the Medisoft menu bar? (Obj. 2-2)

   _____

   _____

   _____

   _____

6. Which menu includes an option to print a day sheet? (Obj. 2-4)

   _____

7. How would you change the Medisoft Program Date to September 8, 2011? (Obj. 2-5)

   _____

   _____

   _____

   _____

8. Why is it important to know how to change the date in a program such as Medisoft? (Obj. 2-5)

_____

_____

_____

_____

Managing Data with a Computerized System

WHAT YOU NEED TO KNOW

To complete this chapter, you need to know:

- Options available in a computerized system.
- Start-up and exit procedures for Medisoft.
- Steps to select menu options.

WHAT YOU WILL LEARN

When you finish this chapter, you will be able to complete the following objectives:

3-1. Define the terms used in this chapter.

3-2. Use the computer keyboard to enter information in Medisoft.

3-3. Navigate the Medisoft data entry windows.

3-4. Search for information in Medisoft.

3-5. Add a new procedure code to a Medisoft database.

3-6. Create a new chart number for a patient.

3-7. Back up your data.

KEY TERMS

Backup data A copy of data files at a specific point in time that can be used to restore data to the system.

Chart number A unique number that identifies each patient, used on all documents that pertain to that patient in Medisoft.

Removable media device A device that stores data but is not a permanent part of a computer.

Restoring data The process of retrieving data from backup storage devices.

Entering and Editing Data

All data, whether patients' addresses or charges for procedures, are entered into Medisoft through the menus on the menu bar or through the buttons on the toolbar. Selecting an option from the menus or toolbar brings up a dialog box. The Tab key is used to move between text boxes within a dialog box. In some dialog boxes, information is entered by keying data into a text box. For example, a patient's name would be keyed directly into a text box. At other times, selections are made from a list of choices already present. For example, when entering the name of the provider a patient is seeing, the provider is selected from a drop-down list of providers already in the system.

Editing Data

If you make a mistake when entering text in a field, use the Backspace and Delete keys to delete incorrect text. Then enter the correct information. The Backspace key deletes characters immediately to the left of the cursor. The Delete key deletes highlighted characters, or, if no characters are highlighted, it deletes characters immediately to the right of the cursor.

Saving Data

Information entered into Medisoft is saved by clicking the Save button that appears in most dialog boxes (those in which data have been input).

Deleting Data

Some Medisoft dialog boxes contain buttons for the purpose of deleting data. For example, to delete an insurance carrier, the entry for the carrier is clicked in the Insurance Carrier List dialog box. Then the Delete button is clicked. In most cases, Medisoft will ask for a confirmation before deleting the data.

In most dialog boxes, data can also be deleted by highlighting the information and clicking the right mouse button. A shortcut menu that contains an option to delete the transaction is displayed. Again, Medisoft will ask for confirmation before deleting the data. A record of deletions is stored in a database and can be viewed in an audit report.

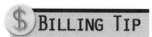

BILLING TIP

Clicking the right mouse button while pointing to a field displays a menu with options to enter or edit data.

✓CHECKPOINT

1. How does the Backspace key function when editing data?

2. How does the Delete key function when editing data?

3. How can you delete an insurance carrier from the database?

Follow these steps to practice entering information and correcting errors.

1. Start the Medisoft program.

2. Set the Medisoft Program Date to September 6, 2010. If an Information box appears saying that the date you have selected is a future date, click OK to continue.

3. Pull down the Activities menu and select the Enter Transactions option, or click the Transaction Entry button on the toolbar. An empty Transaction Entry window appears, as shown in Figure 3-1.

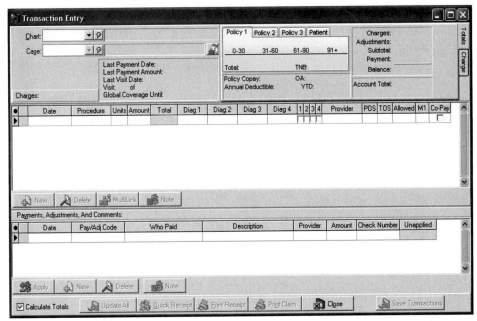

Figure 3-1 *Transaction Entry Window*

4. Key *BE* in the Chart field, and press Enter. Information for Herbert Bell is displayed.

5. Make sure that 2 (Physical Exam) is entered in the Case field. If not, enter the case number.

6. Click the New button in the Payments, Adjustments, and Comments section at the bottom of the dialog box to enter a new transaction.

7. The program automatically enters the date for you (see Figure 3-2 on page 46).

8. Click in the Pay/Adj Code field, and then click the triangle button to display the list of codes.

9. Select 01 (Patient payment, cash) from the list to record a cash payment from a patient, and then press Tab.

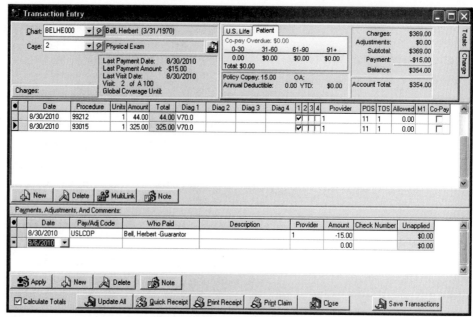

Figure 3-2 *Transaction Entry Window with New Payment Transaction Active*

10. The program automatically enters Bell, Herbert in the Who Paid field, since he is listed as the guarantor in this case.

11. Press Tab to move to the Description field, and key *Cash Payment.*

12. Key *155* in the Amount field, and press Enter. Notice that the program added the decimal point and inserted a minus sign in front of the amount to indicate that it is a payment.

13. Now change the entry in the Amount box to *150.00* and press Enter.

14. Click anywhere in the line that contains the entry you just made, and then click the Delete button.

15. A Confirm box asking whether you are sure you want to delete the payment appears. Since you do not want to save any of the information you just entered, click Yes to confirm the deletion.

16. Click the Close button at the bottom of the window to close the Transaction Entry window.

Patient Chart Numbers

The most important patient information is the chart number (sometimes called the account number). A **chart number** is a unique number that identifies a patient. Medisoft requires that you assign an eight-character chart number to each patient.

- A chart number can include any combination of letters (A–Z) and numbers (0–9).

- No special characters such as hyphens, periods, or spaces are allowed (this applies to all data-entry fields).
- No two chart numbers in the system can be the same.

Medical practices typically use one of two systems for assigning chart numbers, as described below, but Medisoft will automatically assign a chart number using the first system. You can, however, manually assign any chart number you want.

The first system, used by many medical practices and the Medisoft program, does not require special coding for the chart number depending on whether a patient is the guarantor (person or party responsible for payment). With this system, bills are mailed to each patient, regardless of whether that person is the guarantor. Here is how a chart number is assigned in this first system:

- The first three characters are the first three letters of a patient's last name.
- The next two characters are the first two letters of a patient's first name.
- The last three characters are 000.

If a new chart number generated by the program matches the first five characters of an existing patient chart number, the program uses 001 for the last three characters, and so on until it finds an available chart number.

The second system assumes that the guarantor (sometimes referred to as the head of household) should receive the bills for all members of a family. Here is how the assignment of a chart number works in this second system:

- The chart number for all members of the same household must have the same first seven characters.
- The guarantor's chart number must end with a zero.
- Chart numbers for other members of a household must end with the digits 1–9.

As with the first system, you may have to make adjustments if there are conflicts with existing codes.

$ **BILLING TIP**

Most chart numbers end with three zeros (000), not the letter O. Make sure you enter the chart number correctly.

✓CHECKPOINT

Using the first method described for assigning chart numbers, identify the chart numbers that the Medisoft program would generate for these names:

4. William Jackson

5. Julia Hickson

6. Kim Hwang

Searching in Medisoft

As you work with the software, you may need to locate information stored in a Medisoft database. A computer search allows you to find data that match information you have entered, even if you enter only part of the item. Although you may not need to use this feature often as you work through this tutorial and simulation, the search feature is especially useful when working with a large database. Some medical practices, for example, have thousands of patients. Using the Medisoft search feature, you can search for such things as:

- Patient chart numbers
- Insurance carrier codes
- Diagnosis codes
- Procedure codes
- Telephone numbers

The search function works differently depending on the context in which you are searching for data, but the same basic guidelines apply. When searching for a patient, an insurance company, a procedure code, a diagnosis code, an address, a provider, a referring provider, or information about a claim, the Search For and Field boxes at the top of many windows provide a quick way to find the desired information.

Searching for Patients

To begin searching for a patient, you can key the first letter of a patient's last name. As shown in Figure 3-3, keying an *F* in the Search field eliminates all last names that do not begin with the letter *F*, and the selection triangle points to the first chart number that begins with this letter. In our example, the program points to chart number FELST000 (Feldman, Stanley).

As you enter additional characters in the Search field, the program will automatically try to match your entry with the information stored in the database. Using this technique, you can focus your search even if you don't know a patient's complete name.

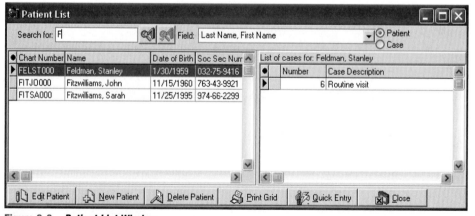

Figure 3-3 *Patient List Window*

The Medisoft program lets you search for patients using any of the following criteria or sets of criteria: chart number; last name, first name; last name, first name, middle initial, chart number; Social Security number; patient ID #2; assigned provider; payment plan; and flag.

Searching for Other Data

The Medisoft program provides the capability to search for data in almost all of its data-entry windows. Whether you need to look up a procedure code that begins with 992 or find a diagnosis code, you can use the search feature to help you locate the information you need. Just enter the information you want to find in a Search field.

Searching for data is not limited to finding information by entering your search criteria in a Search field. The techniques also apply to locating and entering data in a data-entry box. As you begin typing characters in a data-entry box, the program will display the closest match. Then you can use the arrow keys to continue searching in the pop-up list.

> **$ BILLING TIP**
>
> *Since chart numbers usually begin with the first three letters of a patient's last name, you can use this information to help you quickly locate a patient's chart number.*

Computer Practice 3-2: *Searching for a Patient Chart Number*

Practice searching for a patient chart number following these steps:

1. Select Patients/Guarantors and Cases on the Lists menu, or click the corresponding Patient List toolbar button.

2. Key the letter *F* in the Search For field to begin your search for Sarah Fitzwilliams's chart number.

3. The program displays a list of patient chart numbers and highlights the first record that begins with the letter *F* (FELST000—Feldman, Stanley).

4. Continue to narrow your search by typing the letter *I* in the field. As you can see, the program highlights the first patient chart number that begins with the letters *FI*. You can continue to use this method until you find an exact match, or you can simply select the record by clicking it once you see it in the list.

5. Move back to the Search For field, and use the Backspace key to erase the letters *FI*. Notice that the full list of patients is displayed.

6. Use the steps you just practiced to search for and select Hal Sampson's chart number.

7. Practice finding other chart numbers.

8. Click the Close button in the Patient List window when you are finished.

> **$ BILLING TIP**
>
> *Remember to press the Tab or Enter key to move to the next field. If you need to go back to a field, press Shift+Tab.*

> **$ BILLING TIP**
>
> *You can press the Backspace key in a search box to reset the search criteria so that you can begin again.*

> **$ BILLING TIP**
>
> *You can also use the Locate (magnifying glass) button in the Transaction Entry window to find a patient or a case. This button is located to the right of the Chart and Case data-entry boxes. Selecting this option opens the Patient Search window or Case Search window in which you can search for the specific record you need.*

Computer Practice 3-3: *Searching for a Procedure Code*

Practice searching for a procedure code following these steps:

1. Pull down the Lists menu, and choose the Procedure/Payment/ Adjustment Codes option. You can also click the Procedure Code List button on the toolbar. Suppose you want to find the procedure code for a routine moderate exam for an existing (established) patient, but you can remember only that the code begins with 99.

2. Make sure the Field box to the right of the Search For field is set to Code 1, and then enter *99* in the Search For field as shown in Figure 3-4. The program limits the display to codes that begin with the number 99 and highlights the first entry in the list (99201).

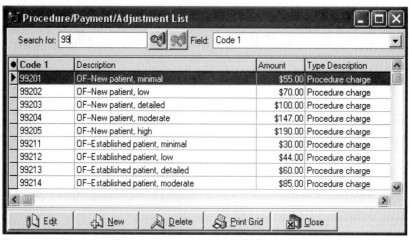

Figure 3-4   *Procedure/Payment/Adjustment List Window*

3. Use the scroll bar or the up and down arrow keys on the right side of the window to scan the list of procedure codes. Did you find code 99214?

4. Find the code for an ankle X-ray. The code begins with 73.

5. Click the Close button to close the window.

Adding New Codes

When Medisoft is set up in an office, commonly used procedure and diagnosis codes are included in the data file. On occasion, however, you may need to add an additional diagnosis, procedure, or other code to the system.

Various codes are routinely used in medical office databases to simplify the data-entry process and to standardize the information reported to insurance carriers. When you add a new code, the information you provide depends on the code itself. For example, when you set up a new procedure code, you must enter the service type, the place where the service was rendered, and the charges for the procedure. The standard Type of Service codes and Place of Service codes are shown in Table 3-1 and Table 3-2. Most insurance carriers accept these codes.

Table 3-1	Type of Service Codes			
Code	**Service Type**		**Code**	**Service Type**
1	Medical Care		6	Radiation therapy
2	Surgery		7	Anesthesia
3	Consultation		8	Surgical assistance
4	Diagnostic X-ray		9	Other medical
5	Diagnostic lab		0	Blood charges

Table 3-2	Place of Service Codes			
Code	**Place**		**Code**	**Place**
11	Office		22	Outpatient—Hospital
12	Home		23	Emergency Room—Hospital
21	Inpatient—Hospital		24	Ambulatory Surgical Center

Computer Practice 3-4: *Adding a New Procedure Code*

Practice adding a new procedure code by following the steps listed below:

1. Choose Procedure/Payment/Adjustment Codes from the Lists menu, or use the toolbar to select this option.

2. When the Procedure/Payment/Adjustment List window appears, click the New button to add a new procedure code. Notice that there are three tabs: General, Amounts, and Allowed Amounts (see Figure 3-5 on page 52).

3. Enter *99402* in the Code 1 field.

4. Enter *Counseling, 30 min., limited* in the Description field.

5. In the Code Type field, choose Procedure Charge if it is not already selected.

6. Leave the Account Code field blank.

7. Enter *1* for the type of service (see Table 3-1).

8. Enter *11* in the Place of Service field (see Table 3-2).

9. Completing the other fields is optional. The Account Code field, for example, can be used in combination with a medical office's accounting system. The Time To Do Procedure field lets a provider include the number of minutes usually required to perform a procedure.

10. Review the information you entered. If you notice an error, move to the corresponding field to correct the error.

11. Click the Amounts tab.

12. Enter *50.00* for the charge amount in Box A.

13. Click the Save button to record the information you entered.

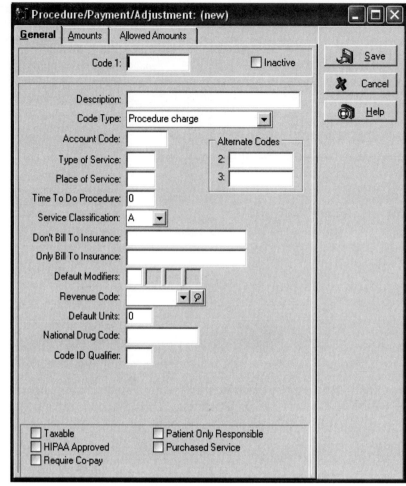

Figure 3-5 *Procedure Code Entry Window*

14. Check the list of procedures to make sure the new code is included.

15. Close the Procedure/Payment/Adjustment List window.

Backing Up Data Files

Backup data files are copies of data made at specific points in time that can be used to restore data to the system in the event the information is accidentally lost or destroyed. In an office environment, you should back up the Medisoft data on a regular schedule, usually daily. When data are backed up, they are stored on a removable media device. A **removable media device** is one that stores data but is not a permanent part of a computer. Examples are flash drives and CD-R or CD-RW disks. Removable media devices may be stored in a location other than the office to protect them from fire or theft.

In an instructional environment, files are also backed up regularly to store each student's work securely and separately. If you are a student working in a computer lab setting, it is important to make a backup copy of your work after each Medisoft session. This ensures that you can restore your work during the next session and be able to use your own data even if another student uses the computer in the interim or if the data on the hard drive have been changed or corrupted for any reason.

In Medisoft, the Backup Data option on the File menu can be used to make a backup copy of the active database at any time. By default, Medisoft also displays a Backup Reminder dialog box when the program is exited. The Backup Reminder dialog box lets you back up your work every time you exit Medisoft. To perform the backup, the Backup Data Now button is clicked. To continue to exit the program without making a backup, the Exit Program button is clicked. The following exercise provides practice.

Computer Practice 3-5: *Creating a Backup File When Exiting Medisoft*

Practice backing up your work when exiting Medisoft.

1. To exit Medisoft, click Exit on the File menu, or click the Exit button on the toolbar.

2. The Backup Reminder dialog box appears, displaying three options: Back Up Data Now, Exit Program, or Cancel. It is best to back up your work each time you exit the program. The current backup file will overwrite the previous backup file (\PBilling.mbk) unless it is given a different name or is stored in a different folder on the computer. To begin the backup, click Back Up Data Now.

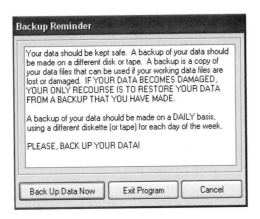

3. The Medisoft Backup dialog box is displayed. Depending on the last time the dialog box was accessed, the Destination File Path and Name box should contain an entry ending with *PBilling.mbk*, the name of the original backup file. You will save the backup file for each chapter to the same place the original PBilling.mbk file was stored, only you will save it under a new name, *PBChapX.mbk*, where *X* stands for the chapter number.

4. Therefore, to back up your work in Chapter 3, edit the filename *PBilling.mbk* at the end of the Destination File Path and Name box to read **PBChap3.mbk.** (*Tip:* Use the End key or the right arrow key to move the cursor to the end of the filename. Backspace over the old name, *PBilling.mbk*, to erase it, and then key **PBChap3.mbk.**)
   Note: Ask your instructor for guidance if you are unsure about where to store your backup files for the course. The instructor may want to assign a specific drive or folder. You can change the path

name to a different location by keying in the new path name or using the Find button to locate a particular drive or folder on your computer. In the following examples, a folder that was created under My Documents called PB7e is used, so that the path name at the top of the Backup dialog box reads C:\ . . . \ My Documents\ PB7e\PBChap3.mbk.

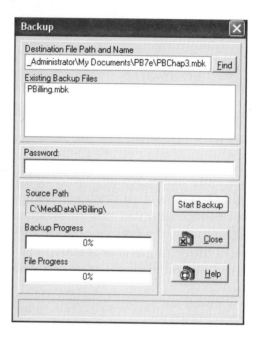

5. Medisoft automatically displays the location of the database files to be backed up in the Source Path box in the lower half of the dialog box. Click the Start Backup button.

6. The program backs up the latest database files under the new name and displays an Information box indicating that the backup is complete. Click OK to continue.

7. The Medisoft Backup dialog box disappears, and the Medisoft program closes.

For safekeeping, copy your new backup file from your hard drive to an external storage device, such as a flash drive or CD-ROM. A separate backup copy protects you from losing your work if the hard drive fails or if you or someone else accidentally deletes or changes data on the computer.

Viewing Backup Data Files

Sometimes you need to see what is actually on a backup disk to answer questions such as the following:

- Is this disk the most recent backup?
- Was the backup process performed today?
- Did the backup run correctly?

If the disk you are relying on for backup has old data or is defective, it won't do you any good. The View Backup Disks option on the File menu lets you see when the backup file was created, the original data path, how many data files are included in the backup file, and the size of the each file.

Restoring the Backup File

The process of retrieving data from backup storage devices is called **restoring data.** When a new Medisoft session begins, the following steps can be used to restore the backup file. A restore is necessary only if someone may have altered the database files on the hard drive between sessions. If you share a computer in an instructional environment, it is recommended you perform a restore before each new session to be sure you are working with your own data.

To restore the file *PBChap3.mbk* to *C:\MediData\PBilling*:

1. Copy your backup file from your external storage device to the assigned location on your hard drive. (Ask your instructor if you are not sure which folder this is.)

2. Start Medisoft.

3. Check the program's title bar at the top of the screen to make sure PB Family Care Center is displayed as the active data set. (If it is not, use the Open Practice option on the File menu to select it.)

4. Open the File menu, and click Restore Data.

5. When the Warning box appears, click OK. The Restore dialog box appears.

6. Use the Find button if necessary to locate your assigned storage folder on the hard drive (the folder used in step 1 above). Locate *PBChap3.mbk* in the list of existing backup files displayed for that folder, and click it to attach it to the Backup File Path and Name at the top of the dialog box. The end of the path name should read \ . . . \PBChap3.mbk.

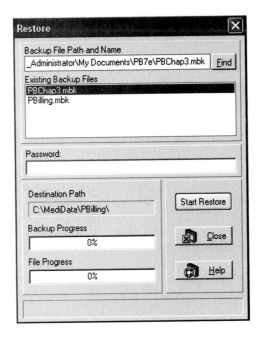

7. Click the Start Restore button.

8. When the Confirm box appears, click OK.

9. An Information box appears, indicating that the restore is complete. Click OK to continue.

10. The Restore dialog box disappears. You are ready to begin the next session.

DEFINE THE TERMS

Write a definition for each term: (Obj. 3-1)

1. Backup data

   _____

2. Chart number

   _____

3. Removable media device

   _____

4. Restoring data

   _____

CHECK YOUR UNDERSTANDING

5. When you enter and edit text, what is the difference between the Backspace key and the Delete key? (Obj. 3-2)

   _____

   _____

   _____

   _____

6. What chart numbers would you create for these patients—John Jackson, Wilma Smith, and David Wong—when it is not important to identify the guarantor or head of household? (Obj. 3-6)

   _____

   _____

   _____

7. What capabilities does Medisoft provide to search for a patient name or other information stored in a database? (Obj. 3-4)

   _____

   _____

   _____

   _____

8. Why are codes used in a medical billing program such as Medisoft? (Obj. 3-5)

_____

_____

_____

_____

9. Explain the steps necessary to add a new procedure code. (Obj. 3-5)

_____

_____

_____

_____

10. What options are available in the Medisoft program to facilitate the backup process in a medical office? (Obj. 3-7)

_____

_____

_____

_____

CRITICAL ANALYSIS EXERCISE

11. You are entering data from Tuesday when a power failure occurs. When power is restored, you find that much of the information in the Medisoft system has errors caused by the power failure. What should you do? (Obj. 3-7)

_____

_____

_____

_____

ON-SCREEN REVIEW

Answer the following questions based on the results of the computer practice exercises in this chapter.

12. In the Procedure/Payment/Adjustment List window, what procedure code is listed immediately before and after procedure code 99402? (Make sure the Search field at the top of the window is set

to Code 1 so that the procedures in the database are listed in numerical order by code.) (Obj. 3-4)

_____

13. What description is displayed in the General tab of the Procedure/Payment/Adjustment window for code 99402? (Obj. 3-5)

_____

14. What dollar amount is displayed in the Amounts tab of the Procedure/Payment/Adjustment window for code 99402? (Obj. 3-5)

_____

Entering Patient and Case Information

WHAT YOU NEED TO KNOW

To complete this chapter, you need to know how to:

- Navigate the Medisoft software.
- Search for information in a Medisoft database.

WHAT YOU WILL LEARN

When you finish this chapter, you will be able to complete the following objectives:

4-1. Define the terms used in this chapter.

4-2. Explain the information requirements for a new patient record.

4-3. Add a new patient account.

4-4. Describe the information needed for a new patient case record.

4-5. Enter a new patient case record.

4-6. Revise patient information.

KEY TERMS

Capitated plan Type of insurance that pays providers a fixed amount for each patient regardless of the actual medical services rendered.

Case billing code A code used to group or organize patients for billing purposes, such as *M* for Medicare or *C* for cash patient.

Copayment Standard fee set up by an insurance carrier that the patient pays to the provider at the time the medical services are rendered.

EPSDT (Early and Periodic Screening, Diagnosis, and Treatment) Well-baby program sponsored by Medicaid.

Established patient A patient who has received medical care from a physician in the practice in the last three years.

Global coverage period Specified period of time during which all transactions for a case with a surgical procedure charge default to a zero charge because the initial charge automatically includes the follow-up work.

New patient A patient who has never visited the medical office or has not received professional care from any of the providers in the office in the last three years.

Patient billing code A code that indicates the schedule of fees that applies to the patient.

Patient information form A form completed by a patient that includes personal information such as name, address, employer, insurance coverage, and any known allergies.

Signature on file Field used to indicate whether a patient's signature authorizing treatment and payment is on file.

Type Field used to identify an individual or another party as a patient or a guarantor.

How Patient Information Is Organized

The Medisoft program requires you to maintain an up-to-date patient database so that the software can process the billing information efficiently. To keep the patient database current, you will need to add information for new patients and update existing patient records. For medical billing purposes, a **new patient** is a patient who has never visited the office or who has not seen any of the providers in the office in the last three years. An **established patient** has received medical care in the office during the last three years.

When a new patient visits a medical office, he or she must fill out a patient information form similar to the one shown in Figure 4-1. The **patient information form** is used to gather personal information such as the patient's name, address, employer, insurance information, and any known allergies. Every new patient must complete one of these forms on his or her initial visit. An established patient may also need to complete this form if pertinent information such as employer, insurance carrier, or address needs to be updated.

HIPAA Tip > The HIPAA Privacy Rule is the first comprehensive federal protection for the privacy of health information. Its national standards protect individuals' medical records and other personal health information. The privacy rule must be followed by all health plans, health care clearinghouses, and health care providers and by their business associates. The rules mandate that these groups must:

- Adopt a set of privacy practices that are appropriate for its health care services

- Notify patients about their privacy rights and about how their information can be used or disclosed

- Train employees so that they understand the privacy practices

- Appoint a staff member to be the privacy official responsible for seeing that the privacy practices are adopted and followed

- Secure patient records containing individually identifiable health information so that they are not readily available to people who do not need them

---

PATIENT INFORMATION FORM

THIS SECTION REFERS TO PATIENT ONLY

Name: Juan Lomos	Sex: M	Marital Status: ☐ S ☒ M ☐ D ☐ W	Birth Date: 7/21/52

Address: 12 Briar Lane	SS#: 716-83-0061

City: Stephenson	State: OH	Zip: 60089	Employer: Stephenson Wire Works (full-time)

Home Phone: 614-221-0202	Employer's Address: 125 Stephenson Road

Work Phone: 614-525-0215	City: Stephenson	State: OH	Zip: 60089

Spouse's Name:	Spouse's Employer:

Emergency Contact:	Relationship:	Phone #:

FILL IN IF PATIENT IS A MINOR

Parent/Guardian's Name:	Sex:	Marital Status: ☐ S ☐ M ☐ D ☐ W	Birth Date:

Phone:	SS#:

Address:	Employer:

City: State: Zip:	Employer's Address:

Student Status:	City:	State:	Zip:

INSURANCE INFORMATION

Primary Insurance Company: Blue Cross Blue Shield	Secondary Insurance Company:

Subscriber's Name: Juan Lomos	Birth Date: 7/21/52	Subscriber's Name: Birth Date:

Plan: Traditional	SS#: 716-83-0061	Plan:

Policy #: 716830061	Group #: 126	Policy #: Group #:

Copayment: Deductible: Price Code: $250 A	

OTHER INFORMATION

Reason for visit: Auto accident--back injury	Allergy to Medication (list):

Name of referring physician:	If auto accident, list date and state in which it occurred: OH -- 8/8/10

I authorize treatment and agree to pay all fees and charges for the person named above. I agree to pay all charges shown by statements, promptly upon their presentation, unless credit arrangements are agreed upon in writing.

I authorize payment directly to FAMILY CARE CENTER of insurance benefits otherwise payable to me. I hereby authorize the release of any medical information necessary in order to process a claim for payment in my behalf.

Juan Lomos	9/3/10
(Patient's Signature/Parent or Guardian's Signature)	(Date)

I plan to make payment of my medical expenses as follows (check one or more):

__X__ Insurance(as above)   __X__ Cash/Check/Credit/Debit Card   _____ Medicare   _____ Medicaid   _____ Workers' Comp.

Figure 4-1 *Sample Patient Information Form*

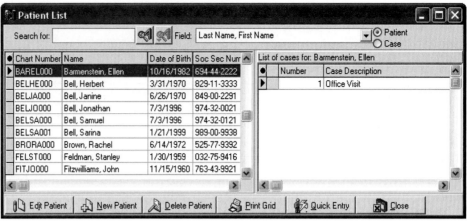

Figure 4-2 *Patient List Window*

Patient/Guarantor Information Requirements

As you can see by looking at Figure 4-1, the patient information form contains a substantial amount of information. Some of this information is used when you add a new patient to the patient database. The other information is required when you set up a new case for a patient. You will learn how to do both in this chapter.

The option to add a new patient is located in the Patient List window that appears when you choose Patients/Guarantors and Cases from the Lists menu (see Figure 4-2). To enter a new patient in Medisoft, you click the New Patient button located at the bottom of the Patient List window. When this button is clicked, the Patient/Guarantor window is displayed with the Name, Address tab active (see Figure 4-3). The other two tabs in the Patient/Guarantor window are the Other Information tab and the Payment Plan tab.

Name, Address   The following fields are listed in the Name/Address tab within the Patient/Guarantor window:

- Chart Number
- Patient Name (Last Name, First Name, and Middle Initial)
- Address (Street, City, State, ZIP Code, and Country)
- E-mail
- Phone Numbers (Home, Work, Cell, Fax, Other)
- Birth Date
- Sex
- Birth Weight and Units
- Social Security Number
- Entity Type

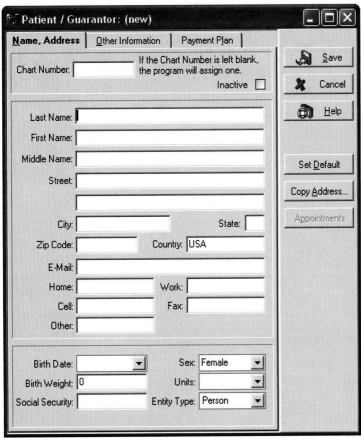

Figure 4-3 *Patient/Guarantor Window*

Other Information The following fields are listed in the Other Information tab (see Figure 4-4 on page 66):

- Type
- Assigned Provider
- Patient ID #2
- Patient Billing Code
- Patient Indicator
- Flag
- Healthcare ID
- Signature on File and Signature Date
- Emergency Contact (Name, Home Phone, Cell Phone)
- Employment (Employer, Status, Work Phone and Extension, Location, and Retirement Date)

Only a few fields are not self-explanatory. The **Type** field is used to indicate whether an individual is a patient or a guarantor. In most cases, you will probably use "patient" for the type. However, there may be instances when the information you need to record is not for a patient. Suppose, for example, that you need to add a new patient account for Mary Lopez. She is a student who attends college in a city near the medical office, but her

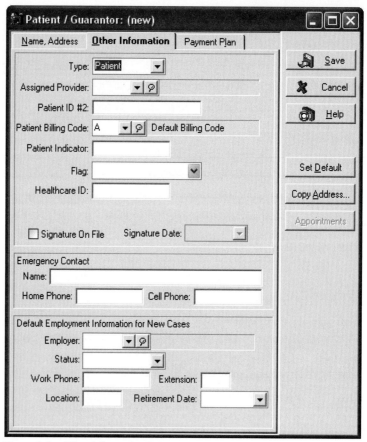

Figure 4-4   *Other Information Tab*

parents live in another state. Mary is still covered by her mother's insurance. In this instance, you would need to set the type to "patient" for Mary and create another record for her mother using "guarantor" as the type. Later, when you enter the case information for Mary, you would reference her mother as the guarantor.

One of the optional fields in a patient/guarantor record is the Patient ID #2 field. This field can serve as a secondary identification code assigned to a patient or guarantor. The code can be displayed in lieu of a chart number on certain reports.

The **Patient Billing Code** field is a user-defined one- or two-character entry that can be used to divide the practice into various groups for billing purposes.

The Patient Indicator field is another optional field. If desired, it can contain up to five characters that identify the patient for sorting purposes.

The Flag field can be used to organize patients into groups and assign a color code to each group. Each patient's record in a given group will be displayed (or "flagged") with the same color when displayed in the Patient List window. For example, all Medicare patient records can be assigned the color yellow, all Blue Cross and Blue Shield records the color blue, and so on.

The Healthcare ID field is reserved for a future national health care identification number as required by HIPAA legislation.

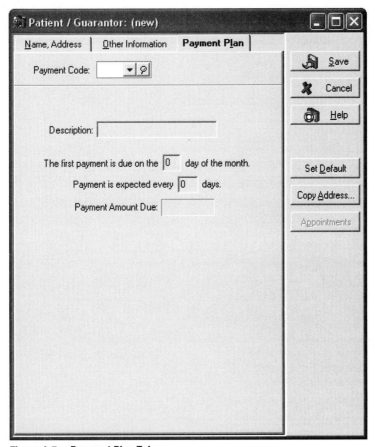

Figure 4-5   *Payment Plan Tab*

The **Signature on File** field indicates whether a patient's signature is on file for authorization of treatment and assignment of benefits.

Payment Plan   If a patient is assigned to a payment plan, information about the plan is entered in the Payment Plan tab. The program tracks the date that each payment is due. If the patient follows the payment plan by making payments on time, the account is excluded from any collection letters that may be sent.

The Payment Code field is listed in the Payment Plan tab (see Figure 4-5). It is where a payment plan is selected. Once you select a plan, the remaining fields in this tab are filled-in by the program. Payment plans are created by selecting Patient Payment Plan on the Lists menu.

Case Information Requirements

In addition to the information described in the previous section, Medisoft stores some patient information—such as marital status, account data, diagnosis, insurance policy numbers, and condition—in case records. The patient case data is organized into eleven different tabs (see Figure 4-6 on page 68). Depending on a medical office's data requirements and the requirements of insurance carriers, a practice may not use all the fields provided.

Using the data provided on the patient information form, you can complete most of the case fields except for those in the Diagnosis, Medicaid/Tricare,

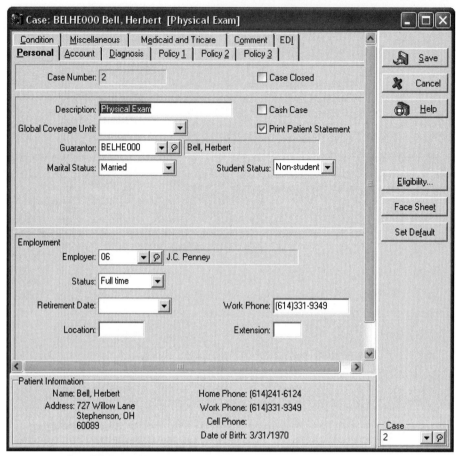

Figure 4-6 *Case Window with Personal Tab Active*

and Miscellaneous tabs. Later, after the provider completes the patient's encounter form, you can use the encounter form to enter the additional information.

A new case should be set up each time a patient comes to see the physician for a new condition or when there is a change in the provider or insurance carrier. When a patient changes insurance carriers, a new case should be set up even if the same condition is being treated under the new carrier. This makes it easier to submit insurance claims to the appropriate carrier.

An overview of the information needed to complete a patient case record is provided in the following paragraphs. Review this information before you continue with the practice exercises.

Personal   The Personal tab (see Figure 4-6) contains personal data about a patient along with the case number, which is assigned automatically. When you complete this tab, you must enter a brief case description or reason for the visit. The tab also includes fields to enter a global coverage period ending date, the guarantor, and the patient's marital status, student status, and employment information. A **global coverage period** is a set period of time during which all transactions for a case default to a zero charge. It occurs whenever a global surgical procedure is recorded in a case. When the initial surgical procedure charge is entered, the charge automatically includes the cost of all associated follow-up work for the specified period.

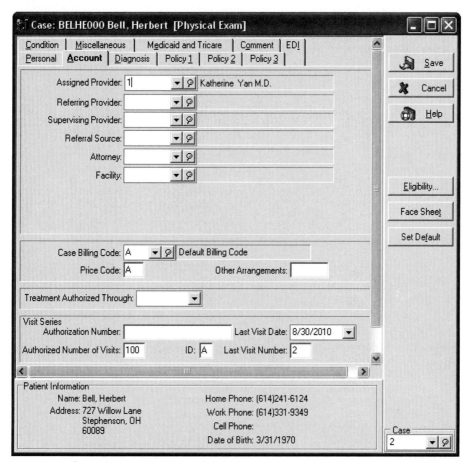

Figure 4-7 *Case Window with Account Tab Active*

Account The Account tab, shown in Figure 4-7, holds pertinent information about the patient's account. Use this tab to record the assigned provider, referring provider, supervising provider, referral source, attorney, and facility codes. Most of this information is listed in the Patient/Guarantor window, which must be completed before a case can be created. The program uses the information from the Patient/Guarantor window to complete some of the fields in the Account tab.

The **case billing code**, which is included in the Account tab, lets you group or organize patients for billing purposes. How you use this code depends on the medical office's specific billing requirements. For example, you could assign billing code A to patients who will receive their bills on the fifteenth of the month and code B to patients billed on the thirtieth.

The price code determines which of the fee schedules is used to determine the amount charged for services. Each procedure code can have up to twenty-six different fees. The fees are listed in the Amounts tab of each procedure code entered in Medisoft.

Another part of the Account tab contains the visit series information. Some insurance companies may require the patient to receive authorization before seeking medical services. A carrier may also authorize a specific number of visits only. In these instances, you can use this area to record the necessary information. The number "counts down" the number of allowed visits.

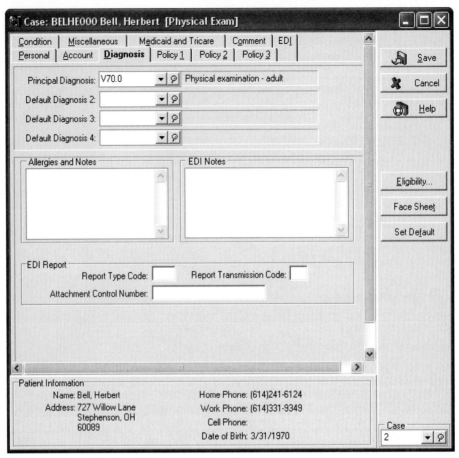

Figure 4-8 *Case Window with Diagnosis Tab Active*

Diagnosis After a provider completes a patient's encounter form, you can use the information on the form to enter the diagnosis code in the Diagnosis tab (see Figure 4-8). By default, you may enter up to four different diagnosis codes. (If more than four diagnosis codes are required, the program default for this field may be changed to hold up to eight codes.) As you may recall, the list of diagnosis codes most commonly used by the office is stored in the Diagnosis database.

The Diagnosis tab also provides space to indicate allergies that the patient may have. The EDI Notes field and the EDI Report fields are used to record information about electronic claim attachments for this particular case. EDI stands for electronic data interchange.

✓CHECKPOINT

1. Which tab would you use to enter a brief description of a case?

2. When you enter a patient case, where should you record a patient's assigned provider or referring provider?

3. Where do you enter a patient's Social Security number?

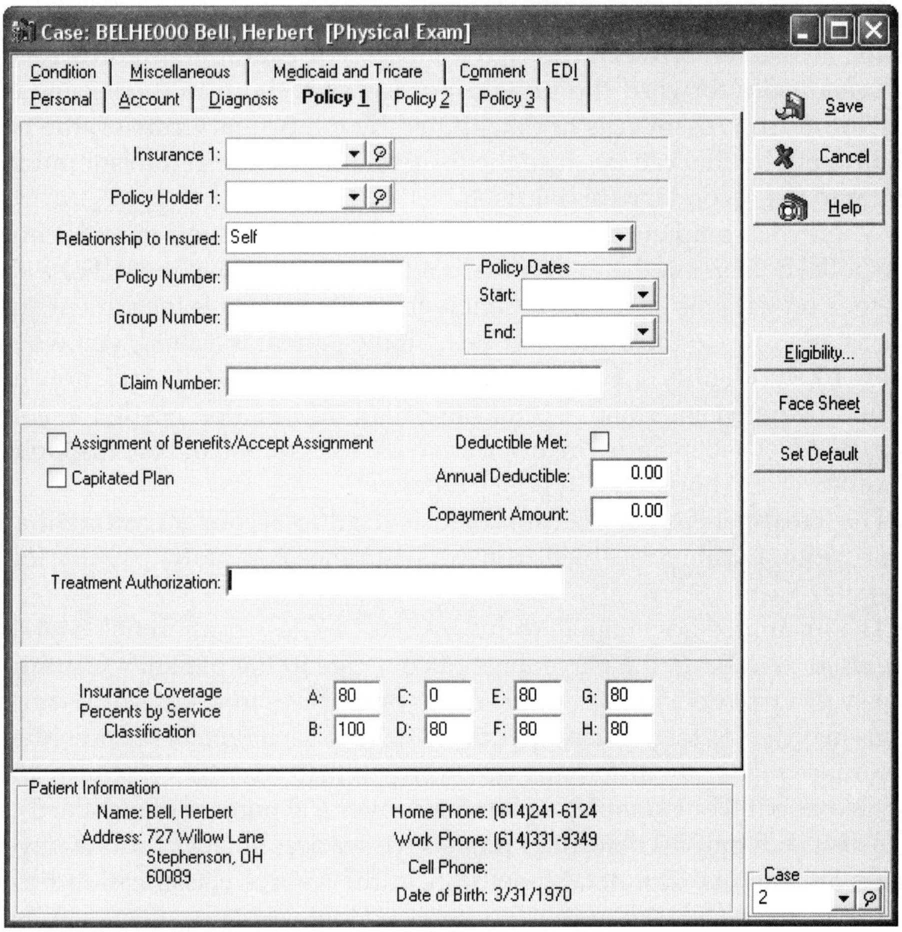

Figure 4-9 *Case Window with Policy 1 Tab Active*

Policy 1, Policy 2, and Policy 3 The Policy 1, 2, and 3 tabs are used to enter the patient's insurance information for up to three difference insurance policies. Although most patients have only one insurance policy, some patients have several different policies with varying coverage. For example, a retired person may be covered by Medicare as her primary insurance. However, she may also have a supplemental policy to cover expenses not reimbursed by Medicare.

Most of the fields in the three policy tabs are identical, except that Policy 1 asks for such additional information as copayment and deductible amounts (see Figure 4-9). Some managed care insurance policies, such as HMOs and PPOs, have patients pay a copayment for each office visit or other service performed. The patient's insurance company pays the remainder of the bill directly to the provider. The **copayment** is a standard fee (usually $10 to $30) paid by a patient to the provider at the time of the appointment.

The Policy 1 tab also contains a box to indicate whether the insurance plan is capitated. A **capitated plan** is a type of managed care insurance that pays providers a fixed amount even if a patient is not seen by the physician during the time period the payment covers. Many capitated plans pay providers this preset amount on a monthly basis.

For the second policy, you need to indicate whether there is an automatic crossover between the two policies. For example, Medicare will automatically forward the unpaid portion of a claim to the secondary carrier. If the crossover is not facilitated by the primary carrier, the box should not be checked because the medical office will need to submit the claim to the secondary carrier itself.

When you complete a patient's policy information, you must identify the policyholder and that individual's relationship to the patient. For a single person with his or her own policy, the policyholder is the patient, and the relationship to the insured is "self." If the patient is a child, you would most likely identify a parent as the policyholder, and the relationship would be noted as "child." Other important information needed to complete a Policy tab includes insurance carrier, assignment of benefits, policy number, group number, and policy dates.

The Treatment Authorization field is used to record a treatment authorization number received from an insurance company, usually for a hospital claim.

The Insurance Coverage Percents by Service Classification fields (A–H) are used to indicate the percentage of coverage in the patient's insurance policy. If a practice chooses, it can group procedures into service classifications in order to assign the proper percentage to each type of service. Many insurance plans pay differently according to the type of service provided to the patient. For example, a plan may cover 100 percent of standard office visits but only 70 percent of preventive services such as routine physical examinations. The default settings in the service classification fields in Medisoft are illustrated in Figure 4-9. However, any of the settings can be edited.

In the case of the PB Family Care Center in this text, because the managed care plans cover 100 percent of all covered services, the settings in Boxes A through H for these plans are always changed to 100. For the traditional fee-for-service plans, which cover 80 percent of covered services, the settings are changed to 80. Medisoft calculates the final amount charged for each procedure based on these percentages.

Condition   You can store information related to a patient's illness or injury in the Condition tab (see Figure 4-10). In this tab, you can include data such as first consultation date, last X-ray date, accident information, and workers' compensation information.

Miscellaneous   The Miscellaneous tab lets you indicate outside lab work and charges (see Figure 4-11). There are other fields to record extra information about a patient. As with other fields in the case tabs, these fields are optional.

Medicaid and Tricare   The Medicaid and Tricare tab is used to record related information such as resubmission numbers, original reference numbers, and effective dates of an insurance policy (see Figure 4-12 on page 74). For patients covered by Medicaid, you can also indicate whether additional coverage is provided by **EPSDT (Early and Periodic Screening, Diagnosis, and Treatment),** which is a well-baby program, or by Family Planning. If

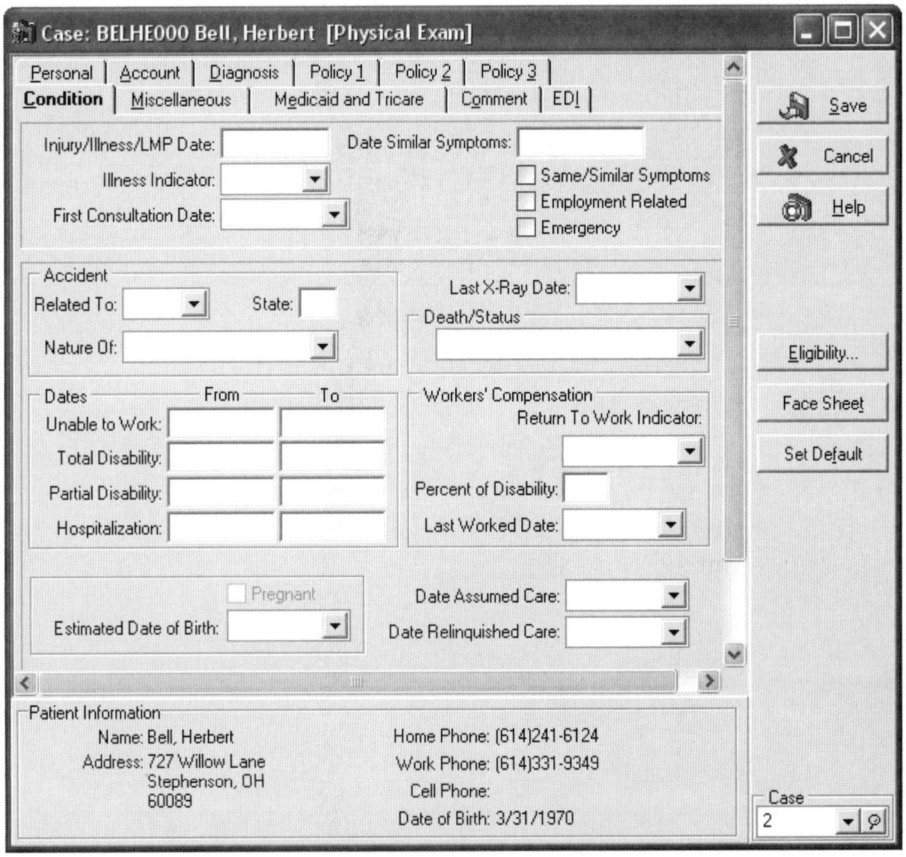

Figure 4-10 *Case Window with Condition Tab Active*

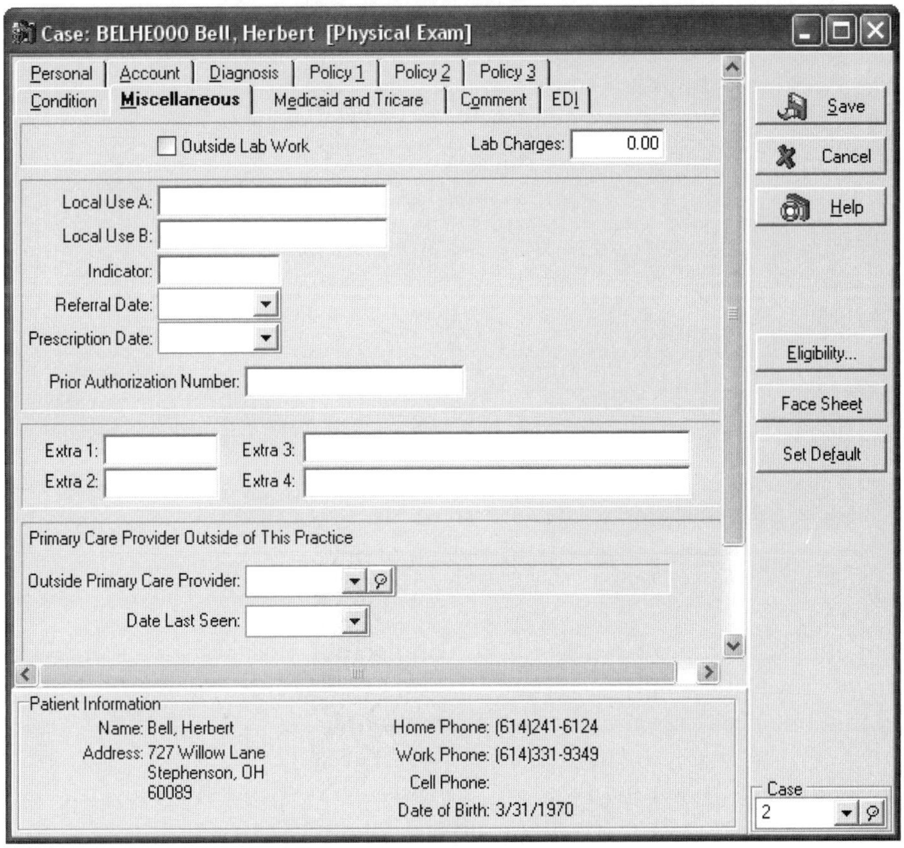

Figure 4-11 *Case Window with Miscellaneous Tab Active*

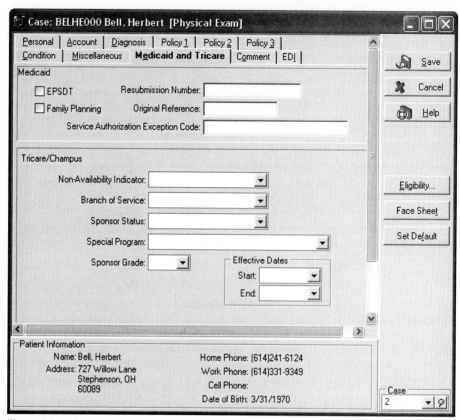

Figure 4-12   *Case Window with Medicaid and Tricare Tab Active*

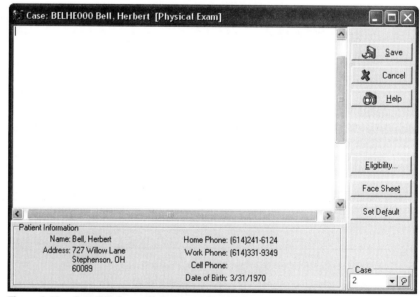

Figure 4-13   *Case Window with Comment Tab Active*

a patient is covered by TRICARE, the branch of service (such as Air Force, Army, or Marines) and the sponsor status (such as 100 percent disabled, civilian, or active duty) can be recorded if required.

Comment   The Comment tab is used to enter case notes (see Figure 4-13). Notes entered in this box will print on statements that are formatted to include case comments.

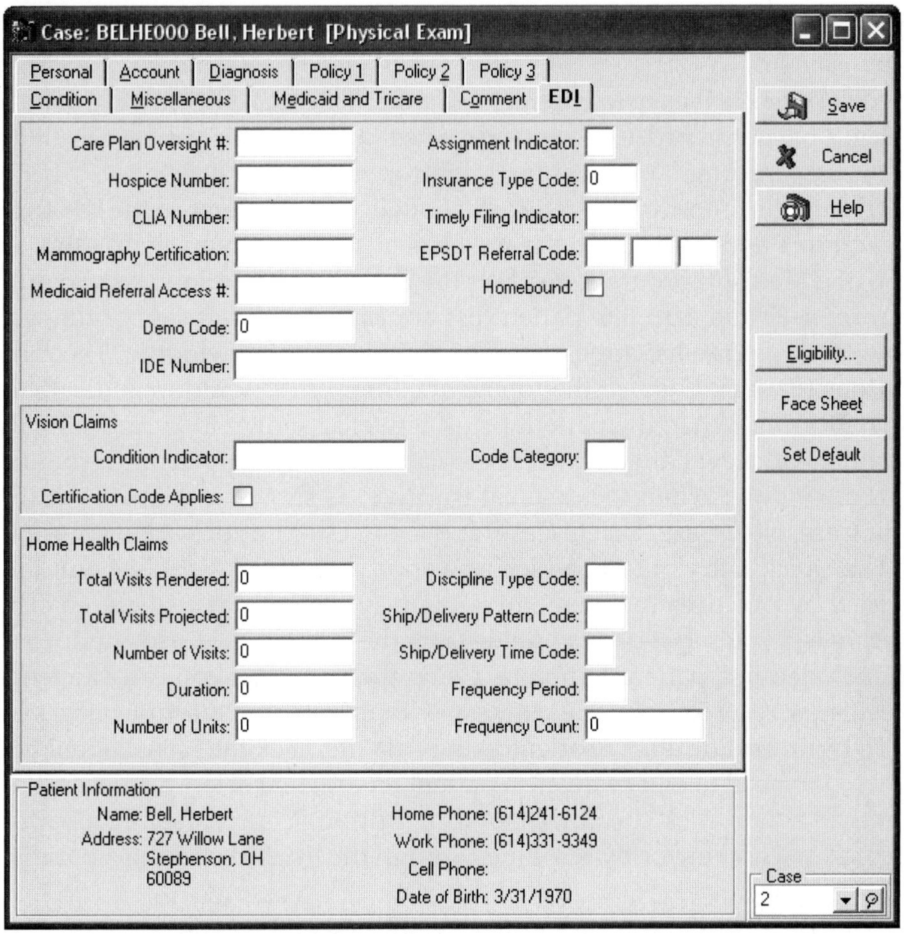

Figure 4-14 *Case Window with EDI Tab Active*

EDI   The EDI tab is used to enter information for electronic claims specific to this case (see Figure 4-14). Only fields that are relevant for the particular case need to be completed.

The top panel in the EDI tab contains fields for entering various numbers and codes assigned to cases for claim processing purposes, such as hospice, CLIA lab, and mammography certification numbers and EPSDT referral codes. The middle panel contains codes specific to vision claims, and the third panel is used to record data required for home health care claims.

✓CHECKPOINT

4. Which field do you use in the Policy 1 tab of the Case window to list the policyholder?

5. Which tab of the Case window would you use to enter outside lab work charges?

6. If a patient is injured at work and receives coverage through workers' compensation, where would you enter information about the accident?

Entering Patient and Case Data

Medisoft makes it easy to enter a new patient record, edit existing data, or delete a patient record. Once you add a new patient to the patient file, filling in the case information is also a straightforward process.

To enter the information you read about in this chapter, use the Patients/Guarantors and Cases option in the Lists menu. When you choose this option, the Medisoft program displays the Patient List window. As shown in Figures 4-15 and 4-16, the patient list appears on the left side of the window, and the case list appears on the right side of the window. The radio buttons (Patient, Case) at the top right corner of the window indicate the current focus. When the patient list is active, as shown in Figure 4-15, the Edit Patient, New Patient, and Delete Patient buttons appear at the bottom of the window. When the case list is active, as shown in Figure 4-16, the Edit Case, New Case, Delete Case, and Copy Case buttons are displayed.

The Quick Entry button, which also appears in the Patient List window, is used by practices that customize the way patient data is entered. This feature lets you select desired fields from the Patient and Case windows to be included in a patient template. Using the template, you can efficiently create new records from one window without opening multiple tabs.

$ BILLING TIP

You can use the Patient/Case radio buttons to set the active area of the window, or you can use your mouse to click anywhere in the desired list to make it active.

To begin adding a new patient to the data file, click the New Patient button. If you need to edit or delete a patient record, first select the desired patient, and then click the corresponding button. You can select a patient record by searching or by scrolling through the list and clicking a patient's chart number.

The case records that appear on the right side of the Patient List window are linked to the selected patient. Unique case numbers are assigned in numerical sequence by Medisoft when cases are created; the numbers cannot be edited. Only those cases entered for the selected patient appear in the list. Remember that you must click the button for the Case list before the program displays the cases.

To work with patient case records, first locate and select a patient record. Then click the Case radio button. If the patient already has a case and you want to create a new case, to save time, you can highlight the existing case and click the Copy Case button to make a copy of that case record. Then

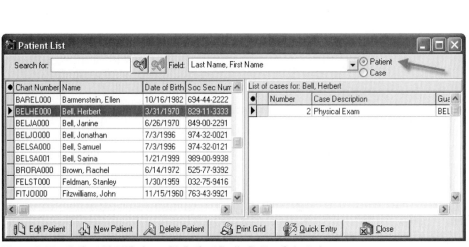

Figure 4-15   *Patient List Window with Patient Radio Button Selected*

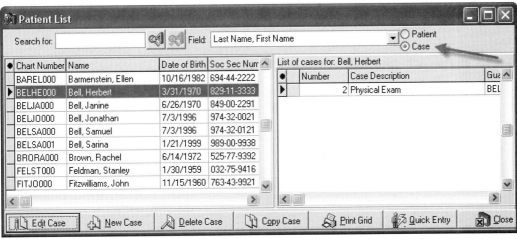

Figure 4-16   *Patient List Window with Case Radio Button Selected*

just make the necessary changes. When you need to edit or delete a case, select it and click the appropriate button.

✓CHECKPOINT

7. Which menu option should you choose to add a new patient record?

8. Which button can you choose to duplicate an existing case?

9. How are case numbers assigned in Medisoft? Can you edit a case number?

10. Which button in the Patient List window lets you change a patient's address?

Computer Practice 4-1: *Adding a New Patient and Case Record (Juan Lomos)*

Follow the steps listed below to add a new patient and case record:

1. Start the Medisoft software.

2. Set the program date to September 3, 2010. (If an Information box appears saying the date you have entered is a future date, click OK to continue.)

3. Restore the backup file you created at the end of Chapter 3.
   Note: Before restoring your data at the beginning of each chapter, make sure "PB Family Care Center" is the open practice. The name of the open practice is displayed on the title bar at the top of the Medisoft screen. If PB Family Care Center is not the open practice, use the Open Practice option on the File menu to select it.

4. Select the Patients/Guarantors and Cases option from the Lists menu, or use the toolbar to select this option (Patient List button). The Patient List window appears.

$)BILLING TIP

- Check the radio buttons at the top of the window to make sure the patient list is selected.

- When you enter the telephone number, don't enter the parentheses or the hyphen. Just enter the number as follows: 6142210202. The software will automatically format the number. The same is true for the Social Security number.

- When entering the birth date, enter the numbers with or without slashes. If you do not use slashes, use double digits to indicate the divisions between the month, day, and year. For example, for the date May 2, 1958, enter "5/2/58" or "050258."

5. Juan Lomos, a new patient, completed a patient information form, which is included as Source Document 1 in the Source Document section at the back of this text/workbook (see pages 183–302). Review the information provided on the form.

6. To add a new patient to the database, click the New Patient button provided in the Patient List window.

7. Using the information on Source Document 1, enter the patient's name, address, telephone number, birth date, gender, and Social Security number in the Name, Address tab. *Note:* You don't need to enter a chart number; the Medisoft program will automatically assign one.

8. Switch to the Other Information tab.

9. Verify that the Type field is set to Patient, and select the assigned provider, Dr. Katherine Yan, in the Assigned Provider box.

10. Verify that the Patient Billing Code is set to A.

11. Click the Signature on File box, and enter the date of the office visit in the Signature Date box.

    Note: After you enter the date, a Confirm box may appear, notifying you that you have entered a date that is in the future and asking whether you want to change it. Click the No button. A warning box then appears, reminding you that the Signature on File date you entered is in the future. Click the OK button to continue. Confirm and warning boxes about the date will continue to appear if your computer's system date is earlier than the dates you are keying in, which, for the purposes of the exercises, are set in the year 2010.

12. Click the Employer drop-down list button. Use the down arrow to scroll to the bottom of the list. As you can see, Juan's employer, Stephenson Wire Works, is not listed. You need to add the employer to the Address list before you can continue.

13. Place the cursor in the Employer box, and press the F8 key, or choose the Addresses option from the Lists menu, and then click the New button. You can also place the cursor in the box and click the right mouse button.

14. Enter the address information for Stephenson Wire Works in the Address window. Use *15* for the employer code. Click the Save button in the Address window to save this new record. Close the Address List window, if necessary.

15. Now you can complete the employer information in the Other Information tab (code, status, and work phone).

16. Review the information you entered in the Name, Address and Other Information tabs. If you notice a mistake, correct the error.

17. Click the Save button to save the new patient information. The program will assign the chart number when it saves the record.

18. Locate the new record you just added. Juan Lomos's record should be selected in the Patient List window. If it is not, click his chart number now to select it.

19. Click the Case radio button or click the right side of the Patient List window so that you can enter the case information for Juan Lomos.

20. Click the New Case button.

21. In the Personal tab, enter the case description, guarantor, and marital status information from Source Document 1.

   - Use the information in the Reason for Visit field on the source document to complete the Description field.

   - As shown on his patient information form, Juan is the insurance policyholder. This makes him the guarantor.

   - Juan's marital status is listed at the top of the patient information form.

   - Notice that his employment information is automatically copied from the information you entered earlier in the Patient/Guarantor window.

22. Switch to the Account tab. Several fields should already contain data that the Medisoft program has gathered from other databases. For example, Katherine Yan should be the assigned provider. Verify the price codes from Source Document 1.

23. Select the Condition tab.

24. Since Juan's visit was the result of an automobile accident, you need to enter this information in the Condition tab. Enter the accident date (*8/8/10*) in the Injury/Illness/LMP (Last Menstrual period) Date field. Place a check in the Emergency box, since this was an emergency. Set the Accident, Related To field to Auto, and enter *OH* in the Accident, State field. Select Injured during Recreation in the Nature Of box.

25. Use the additional information prepared by Dr. Yan (Source Document 2) to complete the From and To dates in the Total Disability, Partial Disability, and Hospitalization fields of the Condition tab.

26. Select the Policy 1 tab.

27. Enter Juan's primary insurance carrier (*Blue Cross/Blue Shield*) in the Insurance 1 box.

28. Verify that Juan's chart number is selected to indicate that he is the policyholder and that the Relationship to Insured box is set to Self.

29. Record Juan's policy information: policy number (*716830061*) and group number (*126*).

30. Click the Assignment of Benefits/Accept Assignment box so that a check appears in the box.

31. Enter Juan's deductible amount (*250.00*) in the Annual Deductible box. Since Juan has met his deductible for 2010, place a check in the Deductible Met box.

32. Enter *80* in each of the Insurance Coverage Percents by Service Classification boxes, since Juan's insurance pays 80 percent of covered charges.

33. Review the information you entered in each of the tabs. Make any needed corrections.

34. Save the case information. When you click the Save button, the Medisoft program will automatically assign a case number.

35. Verify that a case record for Juan Lomos appears in the Patient List window.

Computer Practice 4-2: *Adding a New Patient (Cedera Lomos)*

Follow the steps listed here to add a new patient and case record for Juan Lomos's wife, Cedera. Cedera is also a new patient of Dr. Katherine Yan. Review the information she recorded on the patient information form (Source Document 3).

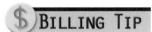

$ BILLING TIP

Use the Copy Address button in the Patient/ Guarantor window to copy an address when entering more than one patient at the same address.

1. Click the Patient radio button, and then click the New Patient button to begin entering the new patient information for Cedera Lomos.

2. From the patient information form that Cedera completed (Source Document 3), enter the information in the Name, Address and Other Information tabs. For this patient, and each time you add a new patient, be sure to complete the Signature on File and Signature Date fields using the date of the office visit.

3. Review the information you entered, correct any errors, and then save the new patient record.

4. Click the Case button, and then click the New Case button to add a case for Cedera Lomos.

5. Complete the case tabs, review your work, and save the information.

   • Enter the information for the Personal tab. Since Cedera indicated that her husband's insurance is the primary policy, make sure to select Juan Lomos as the guarantor.

   • Enter any necessary information in the Account tab.

   • Make a note of Cedera's allergy to penicillin. Enter this information in the Diagnosis tab.

   • Enter the primary insurance information in the Policy 1 tab. Be sure to enter Juan Lomos as the policyholder and enter Spouse in the Relationship to Insured field. Select Blue Cross/Blue Shield for the insurance, and enter the other pertinent data.

   • Record the secondary insurance information in the Policy 2 tab. In this instance, Cedera is the insured party, and the relationship is "Self." Enter the insurance company (*Physician's Alliance of Ohio*), the policy number (*621382*), and the group number (*A435*), and click the Assignment of Benefits box. Enter *80* in the Insurance Coverage boxes at the bottom of the Policy 2 tab.

6. Save the case data.

Computer Practice 4-3: *Adding a New Patient (Lisa Lomos)*

Follow the steps listed above to add a new patient and case record for Juan and Cedera Lomos's daughter, Lisa, who is also Dr. Yan's patient. Review the information recorded on Lisa's patient information form (Source Document 4).

1. Record the patient information for Lisa Lomos.

2. Review your work, and save the patient data.

3. Complete the case information that is shown on Lisa's patient information form.

4. Check the information you entered, and save the new case record.

Computer Practice 4-4: *Adding a New Patient (Angela Wong)*

Follow the steps in the previous practice exercises to add a new patient record and case for Angela Wong (also a patient of Dr. Yan). Review the information she recorded on the patient information form (Source Document 5). Remember to add Peter Wong as guarantor of Angela's account.

IMPORTANT: Angela is a full-time student and is covered by her father's insurance. Her father, Peter Wong, is the guarantor and the insured party. Since her father is not a patient at the Family Care Center, you will have to enter him as a guarantor before you can complete the case information for Angela. The steps to add a guarantor are the same as those for adding a new patient. For the Type field in the Other Information tab, choose Guarantor instead of Patient for Peter Wong.

When entering Angela's case information in the Policy 1 tab, be sure to:

- Click the Assignment of Benefits box
- Enter the copayment amount, which is *$10.00*
- Enter *100* in each of the Insurance Coverage boxes
- Save the case information

Computer Practice 4-5: *Editing a Patient Record (John Fitzwilliams)*

An existing patient, John Fitzwilliams, changed jobs. Previously, he was self-employed. Review the information on Source Document 6. Then follow these steps to edit Mr. Fitzwilliams's patient record.

1. If the Patient List window is not displayed, select the Patients/ Guarantors and Cases option from the Lists menu or use the toolbar to select it.

2. Make sure the patient list (left side of the window) is active.

$ BILLING TIP

If a case record existed for this patient, in addition to changing his employment information in the Other Information tab, you would need to change the employment information in the Personal tab of the Case window.

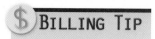

BILLING TIP

As a shortcut, you can double click a case or patient record to edit it.

3. Use the Search feature or scroll through the patient list to select John Fitzwilliams's record.

4. Click the Edit Patient button to edit the patient's data.

5. Switch to the Other Information tab.

6. Change the employment information as indicated on Source Document 6.

7. Save the changes you made.

Computer Practice 4-6: *Updating Case Information (Herbert Mitchell)*

Follow the steps below to update the case information for Herbert Mitchell (see Source Document 7).

1. If the Patient List window is not displayed, select the Patients/ Guarantors and Cases option from the Lists menu or use the toolbar to select it.

2. Make sure the patient list (left side of the window) is active.

3. Use the Search feature or scroll through the patient list to select Mr. Mitchell's record.

4. Once you locate and select the record, select the Shortness of Breath case in the right side of the window by clicking it.

5. Click the Edit Case button so that you can update the case information.

6. Choose the Condition tab, and enter the hospitalization dates shown on Source Document 7.

7. Enter the Medicare authorization number in the Miscellaneous tab.

8. Save the changes.

9. Close the Patient List window.

Computer Practice 4-7: *Exiting the Program and Making a Backup Copy*

Exit the software and make a backup copy of your work by following these steps:

1. Choose Exit from the File menu, or use the toolbar to select this option.

2. Click the Back Up Data Now button.

3. In the Destination File Path and Name box, enter the location where the backup file will be saved (if it is not already displayed). Name the new file *PBChap4.mbk.*

4. Click the Start Backup button. When the Backup Complete box appears, click OK. The Medisoft program shuts down.

CHAPTER 4 Review

DEFINE THE TERMS

Write a definition for each term: (Obj. 4-1)

1. Capitated plan

   _____

2. Case billing code

   _____

3. Copayment

   _____

4. EPSDT (Early and Periodic Screening, Diagnosis, and Treatment)

   _____

5. Established patient

   _____

6. Global coverage period

   _____

7. New patient

   _____

8. Patient billing code

   _____

9. Patient information form

   _____

10. Signature on file

    _____

11. Type

    _____

12. Which tabs in the Case window do you use to enter the insurance information? (Obj. 4-4)

_____

13. Where do you indicate whether an individual is a patient or a guarantor? Describe a situation in which a person would need to be entered into the system as a guarantor, but not as a patient. Can a patient also be a guarantor? Explain. (Obj. 4-2)

_____

_____

_____

_____

14. What is the Patient ID #2 field? How can it be used? (Obj. 4-3)

_____

_____

15. What information is recorded in the Personal tab of a case record? (Obj. 4-4)

_____

_____

16. Where would you record a patient's allergy to a prescription drug such as penicillin? (Obj. 4-4)

_____

17. A patient has Blue Cross and Blue Shield insurance coverage through her employer. She is also covered under her husband's Prudential policy for expenses that Blue Cross and Blue Shield does not cover. How do you enter information on her insurance? (Obj. 4-5)

_____

_____

CRITICAL ANALYSIS EXERCISE

18. A patient has been seen by the physician for hypertension on several occasions within the last six months. The patient's wife just called the physician to say that the patient is experiencing palpitations and dizziness. The physician decides to meet the patient and his wife in the emergency room at the local hospital.

Would you need to create a new case? Do you have enough information to make the decision? If not, what additional information would you need? (Obj. 4-4)

_____

_____

_____

On-Screen Review

Answer the following questions based on the results of the computer practice exercises in this chapter.

19. What is Juan Lomos's chart number? (Obj. 4-3)

_____

20. Who is listed as the policy holder in the Policy 1 tab of Cedera Lomos's persistent cough case? (Obj. 4-5)

_____

21. What is Lisa Lomos's case description? (Obj. 4-5)

_____

22. What insurance carrier is listed in the Policy 1 tab of Angela Wong's Checkup case? (Obj. 4-5)

_____

23. What employer code and name are listed in John Fitzwilliams's patient record? (Obj. 4-4)

_____

Processing Transactions

WHAT YOU NEED TO KNOW

To complete this chapter, you need to know how to:

- Enter information in Medisoft.
- Navigate the Medisoft software.
- Search for information in a Medisoft database.
- Enter patient and case information.

WHAT YOU WILL LEARN

When you finish this chapter, you will be able to complete the following objectives:

5-1. Define the terms introduced in the chapter.

5-2. Explain the information contained on a patient's encounter form and how it is used to record a transaction.

5-3. Enter procedure charge transactions.

5-4. Record and apply payments received from patients.

5-5. Print a walkout receipt.

KEY TERMS

Adjustment A positive or negative amount entered to correct a patient's account balance.

Charge The amount (or cost) of a procedure performed by a provider.

Default An entry automatically displayed in an input field, which can be overwritten.

Inpatient Refers to a patient admitted and discharged from a hospital with a length of stay of one or more days.

Modifiers One- or two-digit codes that allow more-specific descriptions to be entered for the services the physician performed.

MultiLink code A code that incorporates a number of related procedure codes.

Outpatient Refers to a patient who is treated for a medical condition at a facility but who does not stay a full twenty-four hours.

Payments Cash, checks, credit cards, or electronic funds transfers received for medical services rendered.

Handling Transactions

During a typical day, many patients visit a medical practice such as the Family Care Center. The assigned provider performs specific procedures related to the conditions of each of them and records the procedures on the patients' encounter forms. In turn, the billing assistant uses the completed encounter forms as source documents to enter the procedure charges. A **charge** is the cost that a medical office assigns to a procedure.

A billing assistant must process **payments**—cash, checks, credit cards, or electronic funds transfers received for medical services rendered—on a daily basis. Insurance companies send payments for covered procedures on behalf of patients. These payments are transmitted electronically or are mailed to the practice. Some patients make copayments at the time of visits. Others send their payments by mail later, after payments from insurance companies have been received.

On occasion, it may be necessary to make an adjustment to a patient's account. An **adjustment** is a positive or negative amount entered to correct a patient's account balance. An adjustment might be required, for example, if an insurance company does not pay as much as expected and the patient is responsible for the difference.

As you will learn in this chapter, the Medisoft program can be used to process several different kinds of transactions—charges, payments, and adjustments. First, you will learn how to record and enter procedure charges. Then, you will learn how to process patient payments. Chapter 6 teaches you how to record payments from insurance plans, including making adjustments.

Recording and Entering Procedure Charges

For every procedure performed, a billing assistant must make sure that the appropriate information is properly recorded in the patient accounting system. Correctly recording the procedure charges is an important step in the billing cycle. Many of the activities that follow, such as processing claims, collecting payments, generating reports, and managing cash flow, depend on the accuracy of entering charges.

Reviewing a Completed Encounter Form

As you learned in an earlier chapter, the completed encounter form is the primary source of information when a billing assistant records procedure charges. As shown in Figure 5-1, this form includes the provider's name, patient's name and chart number, date the services were performed, procedures performed, payments received, diagnosis, and other information.

ENCOUNTER FORM

9/3/10	**9:30am**
DATE	TIME

Hiro Tanaka	
PATIENT NAME	

Dr. Katherine Yan
PROVIDER

TANHI000
CHART #

Code	Description	
99201	OF--New Patient Minimal	
99202	OF--New Patient Low	
99203	OF--New Patient Detailed	
99204	OF--New Patient Moderate	
99205	OF--New Patient High	
99211	OF--Established Patient Minimal	
99212	OF--Established Patient Low	X
99213	OF--Established Patient Detailed	
99214	OF--Established Patient Moderate	
99215	OF--Established Patient High	
99381	Under 1 Year	
99382	1 - 4 Years	
99383	5 - 11 Years	
99384	12 - 17 Years	
99385	18 - 39 Years	
99386	40 - 64 Years	
99387	65 Years & Up	
99391	Under 1 Year	
99392	1 - 4 Years	
99393	5 - 11 Years	
99394	12 - 17 Years	
99395	18 - 39 Years	
99396	40 - 64 Years	
99397	65 Years & Up	
12011	Repair of superficial wounds, face	
29125	Short arm splint	
45378	Colonoscopy--diagnostic	
45380	Colonoscopy--biopsy	
71010	Chest x-ray, frontal	
71020	Chest x-ray, frontal and lateral	
73070	Elbow x-ray, AP and lateral	

Code	Description	
73090	Forearm x-ray, AP and lateral	
73100	Wrist x-ray, AP and lateral	
73600	Ankle x-ray, AP and lateral	
93000	Electrocardiogram--ECG	
93015	Treadmill stress test	
80061	Lipid panel	
82270	Hemoccult--stool screening	
82465	Cholesterol test	
82947	Glucose--quantitative	
82951	Glucose tolerance test	
83718	HDL cholesterol test	
85007	Manual WBC	
85025	CBC w/diff.	
85651	Erythrocyte sed rate--ESR	
86580	Mantoux test	
87040	Bacterial culture	
87430	Strep screen	
87086	Urine colony count	
87088	Urine culture	
90465	Immunization administration, pt under 8 yrs	
90471	Immunization administration	
90657	Influenza injection, under 35 months	
90658	Influenza injection, older than 3 years	
90703	Tetanus immunization	
90707	MMR immunization	

PB FAMILY CARE CENTER		NOTES
REFERRING PHYSICIAN	NPI	
AUTHORIZATION #		
DIAGNOSIS 848.9		
PAYMENT AMOUNT $10 copayment, check #3022		

Figure 5-1   *Completed Encounter Form*

After a physician completes a patient examination, he or she will mark the procedures performed. As you may recall, the encounter form includes only the most common procedures provided by a medical office. If the physician performs a procedure not listed on the encounter form, he or she writes the procedure in on the form. In these instances, you will have to search for and enter the procedure code when processing a charge.

Most insurance carriers will not pay for treatment without a diagnosis. The diagnosis is the doctor's determination of a patient's condition. Therefore, the doctor must record this information on the encounter form so that it can be included as part of the procedure charge. When you enter the diagnosis, you will use ICD-9-CM codes as the standard way to record this information.

Entering a Procedure Charge

After you review a patient's encounter form, you are ready to enter the transaction to record the procedure charge. You will process all charge transactions using the Enter Transactions option in the Activities menu. Selecting this option displays the Transaction Entry window. As you can see in Figure 5-2, transactions are case-based. Rather than showing a list of transactions for a patient, the program assigns each transaction to a specific case. This means that you cannot enter or edit a transaction until you select a chart number and a case number. Accounting systems such as Medisoft that use case-based transactions allow for much more detailed reporting, which is often required when processing insurance claims.

When you enter procedure charges, you must enter a separate transaction for each charge rather than combining all procedures for a given visit into a single transaction. This step is required because you must provide detailed information about each charge, including a description and an amount.

Once you enter a chart number and a case number, you can enter a new transaction by clicking the New button in the Charges section of the

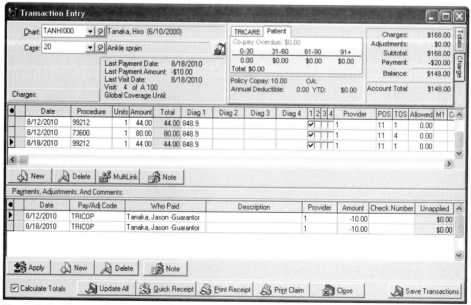

Figure 5-2 *Transaction Entry Window*

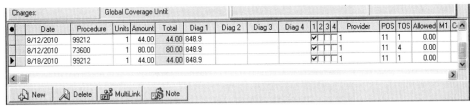

	Date	Procedure	Units	Amount	Total	Diag 1	Diag 2	Diag 3	Diag 4	1	2	3	4	Provider	POS	TOS	Allowed	M1	C
	8/12/2010	99212	1	44.00	44.00	848.9				✔				1	11	1	0.00		
	8/12/2010	73600	1	80.00	80.00	848.9				✔				1	11	4	0.00		
▶	8/18/2010	99212	1	44.00	44.00	848.9				✔				1	11	1	0.00		

New   Delete   MultiLink   Note

Figure 5-3 *Charges Area Within the Transaction Entry Window*

window (see Figure 5-3). When you click this button, the program creates a new transaction line. A **default** is an entry that automatically appears in a field and will be accepted unless you change the information. By default, the program enters the current date (the Medisoft Program Date) and other select information for the new transaction. Usually you do not have to change the default entries.

To record a procedure charge, you must identify the procedure by using its corresponding CPT code. When you enter a procedure code, the Medisoft program automatically fills in the fields based on the information stored in the practice's procedure database. This information can be edited if necessary.

After you record a procedure code, you can enter additional information in the M1 (Modifier 1) field to further define a procedure. **Modifiers** are special codes that allow more-specific descriptions to be entered for the services the physician performed. For example, a modifier needs to be used when the circumstances require services beyond those normally associated with a particular procedure code. A common modifier is –90, which indicates that the procedure was performed by an outside laboratory. If a modifier is indicated on an encounter form, it is entered in the M1 box located at the end of the transaction line. Fields for entering up to three additional modifiers can be added if required.

The Co-pay box, also located at the end of the transaction line, is an optional field that can be used to indicate that a procedure requires a copayment from the patient. A copayment is usually collected at the time of service. Typically, managed care plans require a $10 to $25 copayment with each office visit. If a procedure code such as 99211 (Office visit, established patient, minimal) is defined in the database as a code that requires a co-pay, the Co-pay box is checked automatically when the procedure code is entered in the Transaction Entry window. The box can also be checked manually. The check reminds the billing assistant to collect the co-pay from the patient. In the Family Care Center database, the Co-pay box is not used.

Although most procedures take place in the office, some patients may receive inpatient or outpatient care. **Inpatient** refers to care provided when patients must stay overnight at a hospital. **Outpatient,** on the other hand, refers to medical care provided in a facility when the patient does not stay for a full twenty-four hours. The outpatient facility may be a doctor's office, a clinic, a hospital, a same-day surgery center, or the like.

Use the POS (place of service) field to enter a code that identifies the location for the procedure. The standard numerical codes are as follows:

11 Provider's office

21 Inpatient hospital

22 Outpatient hospital

23 Hospital emergency room

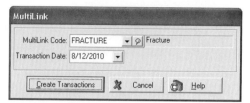

Figure 5-4 *MultiLink Dialog Box*

The Diag 1, 2, 3, and 4 boxes and corresponding Diagnosis check boxes are used to link a procedure to a particular diagnosis. If a diagnosis has been entered in the Diagnosis tab of the Case folder, it will also appear here.

Medisoft provides a feature that saves time when entering multiple CPT codes that are related. A **MultiLink code** is a single code that incorporates a number of procedure codes that relate to a single activity. Using MultiLink codes saves time by eliminating the need to enter related multiple procedure codes one at a time.

For example, suppose a MultiLink code is created for the procedures related to diagnosing a strep throat. The code is labeled "STREP" and includes three procedures: 99212, Office Visit, Low; 87430, Strep screen; and 85025, CBC w/diff. When the MultiLink code STREP is selected, all three procedure codes are automatically entered by the system, eliminating the need to make three different entries. The MultiLink feature saves time by reducing the number of procedure code entries, and it also reduces omission errors. When procedure codes are entered as a MultiLink code, it is impossible to forget to enter a procedure, since all the codes that are in the MultiLink group are entered automatically.

Clicking the MultiLink button in the Transaction Entry window displays the MultiLink dialog box (see Figure 5-4). After a MultiLink code is selected from the drop-down list, the Create Transactions button is clicked. The codes and charges for each procedure are automatically added to the list of transactions in the Transaction Entry window.

After you record and save the last procedure, you can review the transaction data provided in the Totals area of the Transaction Entry window. The Totals tab, located in the upper right corner of the window, displays the total amount of the procedure charges, adjustments, and payments for the current case, a balance for the current case, and an account total for all of the patient's cases. The Charge tab, located in the same area of the screen, can be opened in place of the Totals tab. The Charge tab displays information about who is responsible for the charges (Insurance 1, 2, 3, or Guarantor).

Computer Practice 5-1: *Entering a Patient Charge (Cedera Lomos)*

The encounter form for Cedera Lomos is shown in Source Document 8. Record the diagnosis and the procedure charge by following these steps.

1. Start the Medisoft program.

2. Set the program date to September 3, 2010.

3. Make sure that PB Family Care Center is the open practice, and then restore the backup file that you created at the end of Chapter 4.

4. Review the information shown on the encounter form in Source Document 8. As you can see, there is one procedure charge (OF—New Patient, Moderate) and a diagnosis (473.9) written on the encounter form.

5. Click Patients/Guarantors and Cases on the Lists menu. Enter *L* in the Search For box. Notice that the list of patients is reduced to those with chart numbers beginning with the letter *L*. With the Cedera Lomos line selected, click Persistent cough in the Case section of the window. Then click the Edit Case button.

6. Select the Diagnosis tab, and enter the diagnosis code from the encounter form in the Principal Diagnosis box. Then click the Save button.

7. Close the Patient List window, and select the Enter Transactions option from the Activities menu, or use the toolbar to select this option.

8. In the Transaction Entry window, select Cedera's chart number, choose the case number for this visit, and press Enter. An Information dialog box appears, reminding you that Cedera is allergic to penicillin. Click the OK button.

9. Click the New button in the Charges section of the window to begin entering the procedure charge for Cedera Lomos.

10. Accept the default information shown in the Date field. The date should be 9/3/2010.

11. Enter the procedure code (99204) for OF—New Patient, Moderate in the Procedure field. Notice that the charge amount ($147.00) and other data are automatically filled in when you enter the procedure code and press Tab or Enter.

12. Review the information in the various fields of the transaction line.
    - Verify that 1 (the default number) is displayed in the Units field.
    - Verify that the Amount field is set to $147.00. If not, check that you entered the procedure code correctly. The amount for the procedure is pulled from the program's procedure code database.
    - For each charge, a corresponding diagnosis must be reported. Since there is only one diagnosis in the patient's case information (473.9), the program automatically selects it for this procedure.
    - Accept the provider information (1 for Dr. Yan). Provider information is pulled from the patient's case information.
    - Accept the information in the POS (place of service) field. The code should be set to 11 (Provider's office). POS information is pulled from the program's procedure code database.
    - Accept the information in the TOS (type of service) field. Code 1 (medical care) should be displayed. TOS codes, like POS codes, are stored in the procedure code database.

13. Click the Save Transactions button to save your work. A Date of Service Validation dialog box may appear, reminding you that you have entered a future date. In response to the question about whether you want to save the transaction, click the Yes button.

14. When you save the transaction, notice that Medisoft updates the information in the three panels at the top of the Transaction Entry screen, including last payment and visit information in the left panel; policy, copay, and deductible information in the center panel; and case balance and account total information in the right panel (see Figure 5-5).

15. Close the Transaction Entry window.

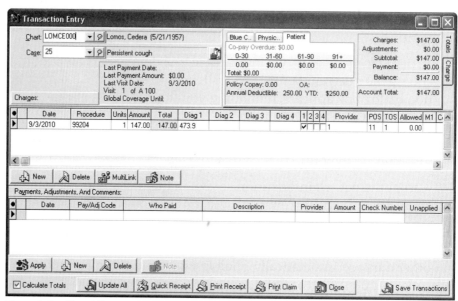

Figure 5-5   *Saved Transaction with Updated Information*

Computer Practice 5-2: *Entering a Patient Charge (Lisa Lomos)*

Record the diagnosis and procedure charge information for Lisa Lomos. The encounter form completed by Dr. Yan is shown in Source Document 9.

1. The date is still September 3, 2010. Select Patients/Guarantors and Cases from the Lists menu.

2. Select the chart number for Lisa Lomos, and open the case for her routine well-child checkup.

3. Click the Diagnosis tab. Enter the V20.2 diagnosis in the Principal Diagnosis field. Click the Save button.

4. Close the Patient List window, and select Enter Transactions from the Activities menu.

5. Select the chart number for Lisa Lomos, and then select the routine well-child checkup case.

6. Click the New button in the Charges section to record a new charge transaction.

7. Enter the procedure code from the encounter form. The program automatically displays the charge amount and other related information from the procedure code and case databases.

8. Save the new transaction.

9. Check your work. The account total should be $140.00 for Lisa Lomos.

10. Close the Transaction Entry window.

Computer Practice 5-3: *Adding a New Case with a New Insurance Carrier (Oxford) and Entering Patient Charges (Leila Patterson)*

Review the encounter form for Leila Patterson shown in Source Document 10. Leila is an established patient who made an appointment to have her cholesterol checked. During the office visit, Dr. Yan performed two procedures. *Note*: Ms. Patterson has changed insurance carriers, so she has completed a new Patient Information Form (Source Document 11). Her new carrier is not in the database, so you will need to enter it based on the information on Source Documents 11 and 12.

Follow the steps below to create a new case with a new insurance carrier, and then enter patient charges.

1. Verify that the Medisoft Program Date is set to September 3, 2010.

2. Click Patients/Guarantors and Cases on the Lists menu. Enter *P* in the Search For box so that Leila Patterson's record is selected in the Patient List window. Note that no cases are currently displayed for her.

3. To create a new case, click the Case radio button and then the New Case button.

4. Complete the Description and Marital Status fields in the Personal tab based on the patient information form.

5. Verify that *A* is listed in the Price Code field in the Account tab.

6. Enter the diagnosis in the Diagnosis tab.

7. Click the Policy 1 tab. When you try to select Patterson's insurance carrier, Oxford, you realize that it is not in the list of carriers. To add Oxford to the database, use the F8 shortcut key to display the Insurance Carrier (new) window. Use the data on Source Document 12 to fill in information in the Address, Options, and

EDI/Eligibility tabs. (You do not need to use the Allowed or PINS tabs.) In the Codes tab, create the Default Payment Application codes as follows: Click in each box, and press F8 to display the Procedure/Payment/Adjustment (new) window. The codes should be named as shown below. Save each code after you create it.

Code	Description	Code Type
OXFPAY	Oxford Payment	Insurance Payment
OXFADJ	Oxford Adjustment	Insurance Adjustment
OXFWIT	Oxford Withhold	Insurance Withhold Adjustment
OXFDED	Oxford Deductible	Deductible
OXFTAK	Oxford Take Back	Insurance Take Back Adjustment

8. After you have finished creating the insurance codes in the Codes tab, click the Save button in the Insurance Carrier: Oxford window to save your work.

9. Back in the Policy 1 tab, Oxford is now selected in the Insurance 1 box. Fill in the other information in the Policy 1 tab using Source Document 11. Dr. Yan accepts assignment for Oxford patients, so be sure to check that box. Also be sure to enter *80* in all the Insurance Coverage Percents boxes at the bottom of the≈window.

10. Complete the new case entry by clicking the Save button.

11. In addition to creating a new case, Leila Paterson's signature on file information needs to be updated. Double click her chart number in the Patient List window to open the Patient/Guarantor window.

12. In the Other Information tab, check the Signature On File box, and enter the date from Leila's Patient Information Form. Save the changes in the Other Information tab, and then close the Patient List window.

13. In the Transaction Entry window, enter both procedure charge transactions for the new case, and save your work. Accept the defaults for the information not provided on the encounter form. Ms. Patterson's account total should be $65.00.

14. Keep the Transaction Entry window open for the next exercise.

Computer Practice 5-4: *Adding a New Case Using the Copy Case Button and Entering a Patient Charge (Ellen Barmenstein)*

Review the encounter form for Ellen Barmenstein shown in Source Document 13. Follow these steps to add a new case and record the transaction for this patient.

1. Verify that the Medisoft Program Date is set to September 3, 2010.

2. Select Ellen Barmenstein's chart number in the Transaction Entry window.

3. A case number appears. Because today's visit is for a different problem, however, a new case needs to be created. Click Patients/ Guarantors and Cases on the Lists menu.

4. Select Barmenstein in the list of patients, and then click the Case radio button.

5. Click the Copy Case button at the bottom of the window. A new case appears, complete with all the information from the existing case. There is no need to reenter all the insurance information; it is entered for you. The only fields you need to change in this case are the Description field and the Diagnosis field. Enter the case description (use "Flu Immunization" based on the diagnosis), and enter the diagnosis in the Diagnosis tab. Save the new case data, and close the Patient List window.

6. In the Transaction Entry window, select the new case, enter the procedure charges, and save your work. Barmenstein's account total should be $96.00. This includes unpaid charges from her August 28 office visit. Her balance for this case should be $52.00.

7. Close the Transaction Entry window.

✓CHECKPOINT

1. Which menu and option do you use to enter a procedure charge?

2. What document do you use as the primary source of information to record a procedure charge?

3. What two pieces of information must be entered before you can enter a procedure charge?

Entering Payments

The next step is the processing of payments received from patients and insurance companies. Payments are entered in two different areas of the Medisoft program: the Transaction Entry window and the Deposit List window. Practices may have different preferences for how to enter payments, depending on their billing procedures. In this chapter, you will learn how to enter payments from patients in the Transaction Entry window. The Deposit List window, commonly used to enter payments from insurance carriers, is covered in Chapter 6.

Patient payments—payments made to the practice directly by patients or guarantors—are entered in the Transaction Entry window. This method is convenient for entering patient copayments that are made at the conclusion of office visits. Insurance payments—payments made to the practice on behalf of a patient by an insurance carrier—are entered in the Deposit List window. The Deposit List feature is more efficient for entering large insurance payments that must be split up and applied to a number of different patients.

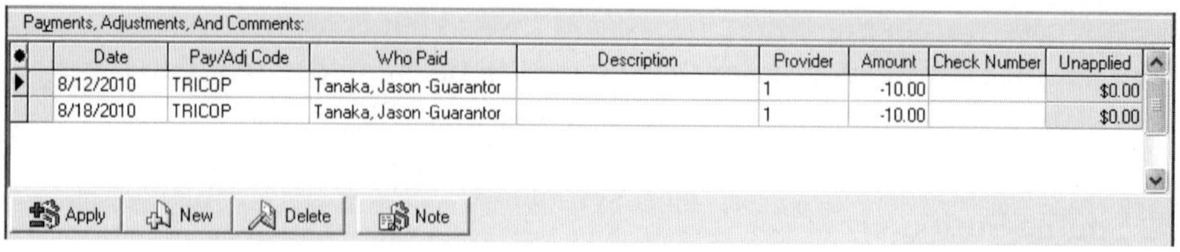

	Date	Pay/Adj Code	Who Paid	Description	Provider	Amount	Check Number	Unapplied	
▶	8/12/2010	TRICOP	Tanaka, Jason -Guarantor		1	-10.00		$0.00	
	8/18/2010	TRICOP	Tanaka, Jason -Guarantor		1	-10.00		$0.00	

Apply   New   Delete   Note

Figure 5-6   *Payments, Adjustments, and Comments Section of the Transaction Entry Window*

Patient Payments

Patient payments, like charges, are case-based. You must enter a patient's chart number and a case number before you can apply a payment to a patient's account. To record a patient payment, you enter a new transaction and complete the required fields in the Payments, Adjustments, and Comments section of the Transaction Entry window (see Figure 5-6). You enter a transaction date, payment/adjustment code, provider, and amount. You must also indicate who made the payment. The payment may be a copayment due at the time of the office visit, a check sent in the mail, or a payment made on a practice's website.

One of the final steps in recording a payment is to apply the payment amount to one or more procedure charges. When the payment being applied is a patient copayment made at the time of the office visit, and several charges were incurred, for example an office visit charge (99214) and an ECG procedure charge (93000), the usual practice is to apply the copayment to the office visit charge before any other charges.

Printing a Walkout Receipt

$ BILLING TIP

To use the Quick Receipt button, the date of the transactions in the Transaction Entry window must be same as the Medisoft Program Date. If the dates are not the same, the program displays the following message, "There is no data available for this report."

After you complete a patient payment transaction, the Medisoft program makes it easy to print a walkout receipt for a patient. Just click the Quick Receipt button to print a detailed walkout receipt similar to the one shown in Figure 5-7. The patient information (name, diagnosis, charges, and amounts) pertaining to the case appears on the printout.

Computer Practice 5-5: *Recording a Charge and Copayment from a Patient (Hiro Tanaka) and Printing a Walkout Receipt*

Review the encounter form for Hiro Tanaka shown in Source Document 14. As shown in the Payment Amount box at the bottom of the encounter form, Tanaka's father pays a $10 copayment with check number 3022 on the day of the visit. Follow these steps to record the charge and payment transactions for this patient and to print a walkout receipt.

1. Verify that the Medisoft Program Date is set to September 3, 2010.

2. Select the Enter Transactions option from the Activities menu, or use the toolbar to select this option.

3. Select Hiro Tanaka's chart number.

PB Family Care Center
285 Stephenson Boulevard
Stephenson, OH 60089
(614)555-0100

Page: 1

7/8/2010

Patient:	Hal Sampson
	3 Broadbrook Lane
	Stephenson, OH 60089
Chart #:	SAMHA000
Case #:	15

Instructions:
Complete the patient information portion of your insurance claim form. Attach this bill, signed and dated, and all other bills pertaining to the claim. If you have a deductible policy, hold your claim forms until you have met your deductible. Mail directly to your insurance carrier.

Date	Description	Procedure	Modify	Dx 1	Dx 2	Dx 3	Dx 4	Units	Charge
7/8/2010	OF--Established patient, low	99212		401.9				1	44.00
7/8/2010	USLife Patient Copayment	USLCOP						1	-15.00

Provider Information

Provider Name:	Katherine Yan M.D.
License:	84021
Commercial PIN:	60-3872-8
SSN or EIN:	810-99-1110

Total Charges:	$ 44.00
Total Payments:	-$ 15.00
Total Adjustments:	$ 0.00
Total Due This Visit:	**$ 29.00**
Total Account Balance:	$ 29.00

Assign and Release: I hereby authorize payment of medical benefits to this physician for the services described above. I also authorize the release of any information necessary to process this claim.

Patient Signature: _____   Date: _____

Figure 5-7   *Sample Walkout Receipt*

4. Since there is only one case for this patient, the case number automatically appears. If there were more than one case, you would have to select the appropriate case to see the corresponding charges. The program defaults to the last case used.

5. Click the New button in the Charges area of the window, and enter the procedure charge from the encounter form.

6. Now click the New button in the Payments, Adjustments, and Comments area to enter the payment transaction. (If an Information box appears with a reminder about the copay, click OK and then click the New button again.)

7. Click inside the Pay/Adj Code box, and then click the triangle button to display the list of codes. Scroll down to select TRICOP—Tricare Patient Copayment—and press Tab. Notice that the program automatically completes the Who Paid, Provider, and Amount fields for you.

8. Record the check number in the Check Number field.

9. Next, so that you can apply the $10.00 payment to the appropriate procedure charge, click the Apply button.

10. The Apply Payment to Charges window appears. In the upper right corner, notice that the Unapplied Box displays the amount of the payment (10.00) to be applied to the list of procedures displayed. Key the $10 copayment amount for the 9/3/10 charge for procedure code 99212 in the This Payment field (bottom row), and press Enter.

$ BILLING TIP

The two buttons at the bottom of the Apply Payment to Charges window—Apply To Co-pay and Apply To Oldest—can be used as shortcut keys to apply certain payments automatically. The Apply To Co-pay button can only be used, however, if the Co-pay box is checked off at the end of the corresponding transaction line in the Transaction Entry window. For the purposes of this text, neither button is used.

11. Notice that the Unapplied box in the upper right corner now says 0.00, indicating that the full amount of the payment has been applied. Click the Close button to close the window.

12. Notice that the Unapplied field in the Transaction Entry window has also changed from $10.00 to $0.00, indicating the payment has been fully applied. Click the Save Transactions button to save the data you entered.

13. Review the information in the updated Transaction Entry window. If you find any errors in your data entry, highlight the field with the error and edit the entry. Notice that the payment is now shown in the lower half of the window. The payment appears as a negative amount (−10.00).

14. Click the Quick Receipt button to print a walkout receipt for the patient. In the dialog box that appears, accept the default selection to preview the report on the screen. Then click the Start button.

15. Review the walkout receipt that appears on your screen. It should list the charge and payment transactions for September 3, 2010. Scroll to the bottom of the window to view the account balance information. When you are finished, click the printer icon at the top of the window to print the receipt.

16. Click the Close button to close the Preview Report window.

17. Keep the Transaction Entry window open.

Computer Practice 5-6: *Creating a New Case, Recording a Charge and Copayment, and Viewing a Walkout Receipt (Elizabeth Jones)*

Review the encounter form for the next patient, Elizabeth Jones (Source Document 15). As indicated on the encounter form, Jones pays the $15 copayment with check number 609 after her office visit. Follow these steps to record the charge and payment information and view a walkout receipt.

1. Verify that the Medisoft Program Date is set to September 3, 2010.

2. Select Elizabeth Jones's chart number in the Transaction Entry window.

3. A case number appears. Because today's procedures are for a different reason, however, a new case must be created. Click Patients/Guarantors and Cases on the Lists menu.

4. Search for Elizabeth Jones in the list of patients. Then click the Case button.

5. Using the Copy Case button, create a new case. Change the entries in the Description field and the Diagnosis field.

6. Save the newly created case, and close the Patient List window.

7. Back in the Transaction Entry window, select the new case for Elizabeth Jones in the Case box.

8. Click the New button in the Charges area, and enter the charge from the encounter form.

9. Click the New button in the Payments, Adjustments, and Comments section. (If an Information box appears with a reminder about the copay, click OK and then click the New button again.) Select USLCOP—U.S. Life Patient Copayment—in the Pay/Adj Code box, and press Tab.

10. Record the check number in the Check Number field.

11. Click the Apply button so that you can apply the $15.00 copayment to the appropriate procedure charge.

12. Enter the payment amount (key *15.00* and press Enter) in the This Payment field to apply the payment to the 99212 procedure code.

13. Click the Close button to close the Apply Payment to Charges window after you record the payment. Then save the transactions.

14. Review the information in the Transaction Entry window. If you made any errors, highlight the field with the error and edit the entry. Notice that the payment is now shown in the lower half of the window. The payment appears as a negative amount (–15.00).

15. Using the steps you practiced in the previous exercise, preview a walkout receipt on your screen. The walkout receipt should list the charge and payment transactions for September 3, 2010. When you are finished, close the Preview Report window.

16. Close the Transaction Entry window.

Review the encounter form for Sarina Bell (Source Document 16). You will use a single MultiLink code to record the procedures. You will also enter a modifier for one of the procedure codes. Sarina Bell's father, Herbert Bell, pays the $15 copayment with check number 309. Follow these steps to record the charge and payment information and print a walkout receipt.

1. Verify that the Medisoft Program Date is set to September 3, 2010.

2. Click Patient/Guarantors and Cases on the Lists menu, and select Sarina Bell's chart number.

3. Create a new case. Complete the Personal, Account, Diagnosis, and Policy 1 tabs. Sarina is single and a full-time student. Since Sarina's father, Herbert, is the guarantor, you can find her insurance information by looking at his case.

   • Make sure to save any information you have entered in Sarina's case before you exit her Case window to look up information in her father's case.

   • Remember to select Herbert Bell as Guarantor in the Personal tab and as Policy Holder 1 in the Policy 1 tab.

   • Remember to enter the correct percentage amounts in the Insurance Coverage boxes of the Policy 1 tab.

4. When you are finished entering Sarina's information, save the case. While in the Patient List window, click the Edit Patient button. Sarina has updated her signature on file information during this visit. Enter the date 9/3/2010 in the Other Information tab. Save the information, and close the Patient List window.

5. Open the Transaction Entry window, and select Sarina Bell's new case.

6. Click the MultiLink button in the Charges area. The MultiLink window appears.

7. In the MultiLink Code box, choose STREP form the drop-down list. Confirm that the Transaction Date entry is 9/3/2010 (if it is not, change the date to 9/3/2010). Then click the Create Transactions button. (If an Information box appears with a reminder about a copay, click the OK button.)

8. The program automatically enters all three codes for the office visit—99212, 87430, and 85025—in the Charges area.

9. Now enter **90** in the first modifier (M1) box for procedure code 85025 (CBC w/diff) to indicate that the procedure was performed by an outside lab.

10. Click the New button in the Payments, Adjustments, and Comments area to enter the $15 copayment. Select the appropriate copay code in the Pay/Adj Code field (USLCOP), and enter the check number.

11. Apply the payment to the office visit procedure (procedure code 99212), the first charge listed.

12. Close the Apply Payment to Charges window, save the transactions, and print a walkout receipt.

Computer Practice 5-8: *Recording a Payment Received in the Mail (Caroline Mitchell)*

Family Care Center received a check (number 3024) in the amount of $60 from Caroline Mitchell for her June 15, 2010, office visit. Since she has not met her deductible, her insurance carrier, Blue Cross and Blue Shield, did not pay the claim. Enter the payment in the Transaction Entry tab.

1. Verify that the Medisoft Program Date is set to September 3, 2010.

2. Select Mitchell's chart number in the Transaction Entry window.

3. Since there is only one case, you do not have to select the appropriate case to see the corresponding charges.

4. Enter the payment using code 02—Patient payment, check. Because this is not a copayment, you will need to enter the amount of the check in the Amount field manually. (Copay amounts from patients are entered automatically by the program, based on the patient's case data.)

5. Enter the check number, and apply the payment to the June 15, 2010, charge (procedure code 99213).

6. Save your work.

7. Caroline's account total should now be $0.00. Close the Transaction Entry window.

√CHECKPOINT

4. Which menu and option do you use to enter a patient payment?

5. Which sequence of menu options and buttons do you use to assign a patient payment to a particular procedure charge?

6. What is the benefit of the MultiLink code feature?

Computer Practice 5-9: *Exiting the Program and Making a Backup Copy*

Exit the software, and make a backup copy of your work by following these steps.

1. Choose Exit from the File menu, or use the toolbar to select this option.

2. Click the Back Up Data Now button.

3. In the Destination File Path and Name box, enter the location where the backup file will be saved (if it is not already displayed). Name the new file *PBChap5.mbk.*

4. Click the Start Backup button. When the Backup Complete box appears, click OK. The Medisoft program shuts down.

DEFINE THE TERMS

Write a definition for each term: (Obj. 5-1)

1. Adjustment

   _____

   _____

2. Charge

   _____

   _____

3. Default

   _____

   _____

4. Inpatient

   _____

   _____

5. Modifiers

   _____

   _____

6. MultiLink code

   _____

   _____

7. Outpatient

   _____

   _____

8. Payments

   _____

   _____

CHECK YOUR UNDERSTANDING

9. What are the steps required to record a procedure charge? (Objs. 5-2 and 5-3)

_____

_____

_____

_____

10. How do you record a payment from a patient? Why is it necessary to apply the payment to specific charges? (Obj. 5-4)

_____

_____

_____

_____

11. To enter a procedure charge, do you have to identify the patient's chart number and case number? What steps are required if a case has not been set up? (Obj. 5-3)

_____

_____

_____

_____

12. What information is printed on a walkout receipt? (Obj. 5-5)

_____

_____

_____

_____

CRITICAL ANALYSIS EXERCISE

13. Why does the Medisoft program organize transactions based on patient cases? (Objs. 5-3 and 5-4)

_____

_____

_____

_____

Answer the following questions based on the results of the computer practice exercises in this chapter.

14. What is the description of the diagnosis in Lisa Lomos's routine well-child checkup case? (Obj. 5-2)

_____

15. What is the cost of procedure 82465 in Leila Patterson's cholesterol check case? (Obj. 5-3)

_____

16. What is Ellen Barmenstein's policy number in her flu immunization case? (Obj. 5-2)

_____

17. What is Hiro Tanaka's account balance after his visit on 9/3/2010? (Objs. 5-3, 5-4, and 5-5)

_____

18. What cases does Elizabeth Jones currently have? What is the balance for each? What is her total account balance? (Objs. 5-3, 5-4, and 5-5)

_____

Processing Claims and Creating Statements

WHAT YOU NEED TO KNOW

To complete this chapter, you need to know how to:

- Enter information in Medisoft.
- Navigate the Medisoft software.
- Search for information in a Medisoft database.
- Enter patient and case information.
- Record procedure charges and patient payments.

WHAT YOU WILL LEARN

When you finish this chapter, you will be able to complete the following objectives:

6-1. Define the terms introduced in the chapter.

6-2. Describe the claim management process.

6-3. Create claims.

6-4. Edit claim information.

6-5. Describe the steps required to transmit electronic media claims.

6-6. Explain how to mark and delete claims.

6-7. Record payments from insurance plans.

6-8. Enter an adjustment.

6-9. Describe the different types of patient statements.

6-10. Create and print patient statements.

KEY TERMS

Claim status The current disposition of a medical claim.

Clearinghouse A service bureau that collects electronic media claims from many different medical practices, formats them as necessary, and forwards them to the appropriate insurance carriers.

Cycle billing A patient billing system in which patients are divided into groups and statement printing and mailing is staggered throughout the month.

EDI receiver An insurance company or clearinghouse set up to electronically receive and process insurance claims submitted by the medical practice.

Once-a-month billing A patient billing system in which all statements are printed and mailed once a month, all at the same time.

Patient statement A list of the amount of money a patient owes, organized by the amount of time the money has been owed, the procedures performed, and the dates the procedures were performed.

Remainder statements Statements that list only those charges that are not paid in full after all insurance carrier payments have been received.

Remittance advice (RA) A document received from an insurance carrier that lists patients, dates of service, charges, and the amount paid or denied.

Standard statements Statements that show all charges regardless of whether the insurance carrier has paid on the transactions.

Claim Management

Claim management is an important activity in the patient billing process. Processing claims involves creating claims, editing them (if necessary), and sending them to the various insurance companies for payment. Claims can be sent electronically or on paper, and the Medisoft program can accommodate both methods. In this tutorial, you will focus on electronic media claims.

Depending on the medical practice, a billing assistant may process claims on a daily or weekly basis. The Family Care Center processes claims on a daily basis. As you work through this chapter, you will learn how to process claims.

To process claims, you will use the Claim Management option in the Activities menu. When you select this option, Medisoft displays the Claim Management window, as shown in Figure 6-1. As you can see, this window includes options to edit, create, print and send, reprint, and delete claims. You will learn how to use each of these options in the following sections.

As you use the Medisoft program, the list of claims in the Claim Management window will continue to expand. Each day you will add new claims to the list of those that have already been sent. Some claims may be marked as challenged or rejected, while others may be held for processing. From time to time, you can remove or delete claims after you no longer need the information.

Creating Claims

After you enter procedure charges, the next step is to create insurance claims. The Medisoft program simplifies this task by automating many

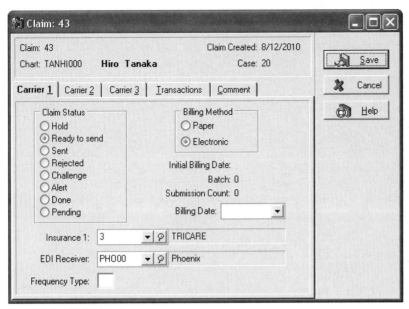

Figure 6-3 *Claim Window*

Editing Claims

You can edit any of the claims that appear in the Claim Management window. Although the claim information generated by the Medisoft program is usually correct, you may have a reason to change some of this information. For example, you could change the status of a specific claim from Sent to Rejected if the claim has been rejected by an insurance carrier. Or you could select a different insurance carrier if this information was incorrectly recorded in a patient's case.

To edit a claim, simply highlight the claim and click the Edit button. When you choose to edit a claim, the Medisoft program displays the Claim window as shown in Figure 6-3. As you can see, you can change the claim status, billing method, billing date, insurance carrier, and EDI receiver for any of the carriers. Using the Transactions or Comment tabs in this window, you can also view the transactions associated with a claim or attach a comment.

Computer Practice 6-2: *Editing Claims*

Follow the steps listed here to learn how you can review and edit the information stored for a claim.

1. Verify that the program date is set to September 3, 2010.

2. Select (highlight) any one of the claims shown in the Claim Management window.

3. Click the Edit button to view the claim you chose.

4. Review the information in the Carrier 1, Carrier 2, and Carrier 3 tabs by clicking the corresponding tab, but do not change any of the data.

5. Click the Transactions tab to review the transaction data for the claim.

6. Click the Cancel button to close the Claim window.

Proofing Claims Using the List Only Option

As the list of previously sent claims grows, it can be difficult to verify the new claims to be sent. The List Only feature is useful in proofing new claims. You can use this option to list only those claims created on a certain date or to be sent to a specific carrier. After you use this option, you should always select it again and reset the criteria to the defaults so that all the claims appear in the Claim Management window.

Computer Practice 6-3: *Reviewing Insurance Claims*

Learn how to use the List Only option to review insurance claims before you send them. Follow the steps provided here.

1. Verify that the program date is set to September 3, 2010.

2. In the Claim Management window, click the List Only button.

3. In the Insurance Carrier field, select 4—Blue Cross/Blue Shield, and click the Apply button.

4. You should see only those claims that match the criteria you set. Notice that the Carrier 1 column displays 4 (Blue Cross/Blue Shield) for each claim. In this instance, you set only one List Only option. However, you could have selected several different criteria to fine-tune your search.

5. Before you continue, you need to reset the List Only options so that all the claims appear again. Click the List Only button again to display the List Only Claims That Match window. Click the Defaults button to reset all the options.

6. Notice that the Defaults button also adds a check in the Exclude Done check box under Claim Status. By default, Medisoft excludes Done claims—claims that have already been sent and paid by the insurance carriers—from being displayed in the Claim Management window. Although these claims are stored in the database, they are not listed with the other claims unless the default is changed and the Exclude Done check box is unchecked. Click the Apply button.

7. Verify that the original list of claims appears in the window.

Transmitting Electronic Claims

In an actual office setting, the electronic claims that you created in Computer Practice 6-1 would be sent to the clearinghouse or insurance carrier. The steps in Computer Practice 6-4 below describe how electronic claims are transmitted in Medisoft. Because schools are not set up to transmit clams electronically, you will not be able to carry out the steps in the exercise after step 3. Simply read through the remaining steps to learn how the procedure would be carried out in Medisoft.

Learn about the steps that you would follow to transmit electronic claims in Medisoft.

1. With the Claim Management window still open, click the Print/Send button.

2. In the Print/Send Claims window, click the Electronic button to change the billing method to electronic.

3. In the Electronic Claim Receiver box, select PH000 (Phoenix). Click the OK button.

   Note: A Program Disabled message may appear at this point because you are not set up to transmit electronic media claims in Medisoft from your location. (Medisoft provides a thirty-day trial period to experiment with the Phoenix electronic claim receiver option. After 30 days, you must obtain and register the program or it becomes disabled). If this message appears, simply click the Exit Program button to close the message box, and continue reading through the remaining steps without attempting to carry them out. Illustrations are provided so that you can understand the process without having to use the software.

4. The ANSI X12 dialog box is displayed, with PHX (Phoenix) displayed as the receiver (see Figure 6-4).

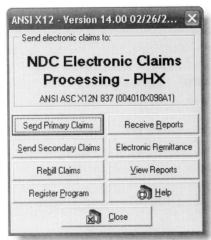

Figure 6-4 *ANSI X12 Dialog Box for Sending Electronic Claims*

5. To send primary claims, the Send Primary Claims Now button is clicked.

6. A Data Selection Questions window appears with various range boxes for filtering the claims. You can choose to send all claims that are ready by leaving the range boxes empty, or you can choose to send claims for a range of patients, a date created range, a billing code range, for a particular provider, or for a particular insurance carrier. Once these selections are made, the OK button is clicked.

PB Family Care Center
EDI Primary Insurance Verification
EDI Batch Verification Report

Claim #	Chart#	Patient Name		Policy#		Group#	Referring Provider	Facility	
	Date From	Proc. Code	Modifiers	Pos	Tos	Units	Diagnoses		Amount

EDI Receiver: Phoenix (PHO00)
File name: C:\MediData\PBILLING\EMC\15.TCH

Provider: Katherine Yan (1)   Group Control Number Suffix: 1

40	WONJO000	Jo Wong		697113321H			Not Found	Not Found	
	Insurance Carrier: Medicare (1)								
	Diagnoses: 1: V65.5	Normal state - patient fear unfounded							
	07/29/2010	45380		11	1	1	Diagnosis: 1		$1,030.00
							Claim 40 Total:		$1,030.00
54	BELSA001	Sarina Bell		50632		6209	Not Found	Not Found	
	Insurance Carrier: U.S. Life (10)								
	Diagnoses: 1: 034.0	Strep sore throat							
	09/03/2010	99212		11	1	1	Diagnosis: 1		$44.00
	09/03/2010	87430		11		1	Diagnosis: 1		$32.00
	09/03/2010	85025	90	11		1	Diagnosis: 1		$25.00
							Claim 54 Total:		$101.00
55	JONEL000	Elizabeth Jones		67339		H344	Not Found	Not Found	
	Insurance Carrier: U.S. Life (10)								
	Diagnoses: 1: 461.9	Acute sinusitis							
	09/03/2010	99212		11	1	1	Diagnosis: 1		$44.00
							Claim 55 Total:		$44.00
58	PATLE000	Leila Patterson		L813229549			Not Found	Not Found	
	Insurance Carrier: Oxford (13)								
	Diagnoses: 1: 272.0	Hypercholesterolemia							
	09/03/2010	99212		11	1	1	Diagnosis: 1		$44.00
	09/03/2010	82465		11	5	1	Diagnosis: 1		$21.00
							Claim 58 Total:		$65.00
47	TANHI000	Hiro Tanaka		13837739			Not Found	Not Found	
	Insurance Carrier: TRICARE (3)								
	Diagnoses: 1: 848.9	Sprain or strain (no site)							
	08/18/2010	99212		11	1	1	Diagnosis: 1		$44.00

Figure 6-5 *Sample Page from an Electronic Claims Verification Report*

7. An Information dialog box appears, asking whether to display the Verification report. If Yes is selected, the Preview Report window appears with a copy of a batch verification report displayed. As illustrated in Figure 6-5, the report displays the details of each claim in the batch. Verification reports may be several pages long. The report may also be printed by clicking the printer icon at the top of the preview window.

8. When you have finished viewing and/or printing the report, the preview window is closed and an Information dialog box appears, asking if you want to continue with the transmission.

9. If you were in a medical office and wanted to transmit the claims at this point, you would click the Yes button, and the claims would be sent from your computer to a computer at the clearinghouse. If you did not want to send the claims, you would click the No button and then close the ANSI X12 dialog box to end the electronic claims processing procedure.

Electronic Claim Edits

After an electronic claim is transmitted, the clearinghouse sends back a claim submission report, indicating that the claim file has been received. The clearinghouse then performs an edit—a check to see that all necessary information is included in the claim file. After the edit is complete, an audit/edit report is sent from the clearinghouse to the practice. This report lists any problems that need to be corrected before the claim can be sent to the health plan. Any claims that require correction have to be resubmitted to the clearinghouse.

After a claim passes the necessary edits at the clearinghouse, it is ready to be sent to the appropriate payer. The clearinghouse transmits the claim file to the payer, and the payer sends back a transmission report. The appearance of this report varies from payer to payer, but the report usually includes the following information:

- Date the report was run
- Payer name
- Provider ID number
- Claim acceptance/rejection status
- If claim is rejected, location in the claim that is causing the rejection

Based on the payer's decision in the report, the payer sends a remittance advice and payment for the claim. After the payment is entered in the database, Medisoft displays the claim status as Done.

Printing Insurance Claim Forms

Occasionally, it is necessary to print and mail some claims rather than transmit them electronically. To print a claim, you first must determine whether the claim is listed as electronic or paper in the Claim Management window. If it is listed as EDI, you will need to edit the claim and change the billing method to paper in order to print the claim. Then you will be able to print the claim using the same Print/Send button that you would use to send electronic claims.

You must also select the appropriate CMS-1500 report format. There are several different CMS report options from which to choose. Some have minor variations that are required to accommodate different printers. Other CMS report options are available to process Medicare claims. For our purposes, always use the CMS-1500 (Primary) report—or, if you have

> **$ BILLING TIP**
>
> *When sending a claim electronically, an attachment that needs to accompany the claim, such as radiology films, must be referred to in the claim. In Medisoft, the EDI Report area within the Diagnosis tab of the Case window is used to indicate that an attachment will accompany the claim and how the attachment will be transmitted.*

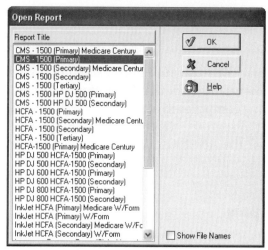

Figure 6-6   *Open Report Window with the CMS-1500 (Primary) Report Format Selected*

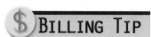

$ BILLING TIP

If you have a laser printer, the Laser CMS (Primary) W/Form option in the Open Report window can be used to print the claim data and form together. This option is useful for proofreading or viewing a completed claim form in the preview window even if you do not have a laser printer.

a laser printer, the Laser CMS (Primary) W/Form report—in the Open Report window (see Figure 6-6).

For most of the CMS report options, other than those that specify "W/Form" in the report title, when you preview a report on screen or print the claim on a blank sheet of paper, the data may not seem to be formatted properly. Remember that a medical office using a paper claim would print the claim on a blank CMS-1500 form to send it to the insurance carrier. The location of the data on a sheet of paper corresponds to the required fields on the preprinted CMS form. For the purposes of the exercises in this text, blank CMS-1500 claim forms are available at the book's Online Learning Center (www.mhhe.com/patientbilling7e).

Once a claim has been printed (or transmitted electronically), the Medisoft program automatically changes the claim status from Ready to Send to Sent. To reprint a claim with a Sent status, the Reprint Claim button in the Claim Management window is used. The claim can be reprinted any number of times, using any of the available report formats.

Computer Practice 6-5: *Printing Insurance Claims*

Follow the instructions provided below to print insurance claim forms for patients whose last names begin with the letter *B*. Since all insurance claims in this text/workbook are set up to be transmitted electronically, you will need to change the billing method for the claims you want to print to Paper for the purposes of this exercise.

1. Verify that the program date is set to September 3, 2010.

2. Open the Claim Management window, and change the Sort By field from Claim Number to Chart Number so that the claims are listed alphabetically.

3. In the Claim Management window, select the claim for the first patient whose last name begins with *B*, and click the Edit button.

4. Change the Billing Method from Electronic to Paper, and click the Save button.

5. Click the Print/Send button. Make sure that you have selected the option to print claims using the paper billing method. Click the OK button to continue.

6. In the Open Report window, choose the CMS-1500 (Primary) report or the Laser CMS (Primary) W/Form report, depending on your printer. (*Note:* If you do not have a laser printer and want to use preprinted CMS-1500 claim forms, insert the forms in your printer at this time.)

7. Click the OK button.

8. Choose to preview the report on the screen, and click Start.

9. Accept the default settings (in this case, all the settings are blank by default) in the Data Selection Questions window, and click OK.

10. Review the claim on screen. If you selected the laser report option, you will see the claim data and the form together. Otherwise, only the claim data will appear in the preview window.

11. Click the printer icon at the top of the window to print the claim unless you are instructed otherwise. (*Note:* If you do not actually print the claim, the claim status will not change from Ready to Send to Sent.)

12. Close the report window.

13. Review the status of the claim. Notice it has changed from Ready to Send to Sent.

14. Repeat these steps to print claims for the other patients whose last names begin with *B*. Remember to edit the claims first in order to change the billing method from electronic to paper.

15. Close the Claim Management window.

Changing the Claim Status Manually

As illustrated in the previous exercise, when you print or transmit claims, the software automatically changes the status from Ready to Send to Sent. For the purposes of this text/workbook, since it is not possible to actually transmit electronic claims during the exercises, whenever you send an electronic claim, you will need to update the claim status manually from Ready to Send to Sent. In the next exercise, you practice doing this with an earlier batch of claims in the database that have a status of Ready to Send.

Computer Practice 6-6: *Changing the Status of Claims*

Change the claim status for claims with batch number 0 from Ready to Send to Sent.

1. In the Claim Management window, click the Change Status button. The Change Claim Status/Billing Method window appears.

2. Click the Batch radio button, and enter *0* in the box on the right.

3. Select Ready to Send in the Status From column.

4. Select Sent in the Status To column.

5. Click the OK button. The window closes, and the Claim Management window reappears with the Claim Status column for claims with Batch number 0 now displaying Sent. Earlier, the batch 0 claims displayed a Ready to Send status.

6. Scroll through the list of claims and note that all the claims now have a status of Sent—the three paper claims that you printed as well as the electronic batch 0 claims for which you changed the status just now.

7. Close the Claim Management window.

Deleting Claims

Using the Claim Management functions, you can delete claims that are no longer needed so that the list of claims is more manageable. Although many medical practices leave Sent claims active for quite some time, you can remove the old claims that have been sent and paid by insurance carriers. These claims are assigned a status of Done in Medisoft. For our purposes, you should not need to delete any claims that you create.

What if you accidentally create claims that should not be included in the list? Rather than delete the claims, you could mark them as Hold. This method is preferable to deleting the claims.

✓CHECKPOINT

1. Which menu contains the Claim Management feature?

2. What status is assigned to a claim before it is printed or sent?

3. After a claim is transmitted, what status does Medisoft assign to the claim?

4. After an insurance company pays a claim, what status does Medisoft assign to the claim?

Insurance Payments

Information about payments from insurance carriers is mailed or is electronically transmitted to a physician as an electronic remittance advice (ERA). A **remittance advice (RA)** lists patients, dates of service, charges, and the amount paid or denied by the insurance carrier. Most RAs also provide explanations of unpaid charges. Sometimes a paper check is attached to the RA; in other cases, the payment is deposited directly in the practice's bank account.

HIPAA Tip **>** Although similar information is featured on the ERA and the paper RA, the ERA offers additional data not available on a paper RA. The ERA that is mandated for use by HIPAA is called the ASC X12 835 Remittance Advice Transaction, or simply the 835. In addition to physicians, other health care providers receiving the 835 include hospitals, nursing homes, laboratories, and dentists.

Understanding the RA

The amount the insurance carrier agrees to pay for each procedure, as listed on an RA, depends on the type of insurance plan the patient has. In the Family Care Center in this text/workbook, two types of fee structures are used—one for traditional plans and another for managed care plans.

In the traditional plans, which include Blue Cross and Blue Shield and Oxford, after the patient pays a deductible, the payer pays 80 percent of the approved charges, and the patient is responsible for the remaining 20 percent. In the examples used in this text/workbook, the provider's fee for each procedure is the same as the insurance plan's allowed amount. Given a $44.00 office visit for procedure code 99212, the provider would receive 80 percent of $44.00 ($35.20) from the insurance carrier and would charge the patient the remaining 20 percent ($8.80). The RA would list the following information:

Proc Code	Amount Charged	Allowed Amount	Amt Paid. Provider	Patient Balance
99212	44.00	44.00	35.20	8.80

In managed care plans, a different fee structure is used. In contracts with managed care plans, providers generally negotiate lower fees in exchange for the advantages of being in the managed care network, such as the possibility of seeing more patients. Often, charges for individual procedure codes are negotiated on a code by code basis.

In the case of the managed care examples at the Family Care Center, which include TRICARE, US Life, and Physician's Choice Services, the insurance company has agreed to pay the provider 90 percent of the provider's charges for all procedures (referred to on the RA as the allowed amount). Rather than bill the patient for the remaining 10 percent of the charge, the provider records the remaining 10 percent as an adjustment. The adjustment is then written off (absorbed) by the provider. The patient's responsibility is to pay the monthly premium to the plan as well as a $10 or $15 copay (depending on the plan) to the provider at the time of the visit. The patient's copay is counted towards the allowed amount. This means the insurance company pays 90 percent of the charge minus the patient's copay amount. In the $44.00 office visit example above, the RA would therefore list the following information:

Proc Code	Amount Charged	Allowed Amount	Copay	Amt Paid Provider	Patient Balance	Adj
99212	44.00	39.60	10.00	29.60	.00	−4.40

As you will see from the computer practice exercises in this chapter, one of the greatest advantages in using a computerized patient billing program is that the program performs the calculations involved in processing insurance payments for you. As long as insurance payments are entered correctly, the program will keep track of what each patient owes after the payment is recorded, based on the patient's insurance information in the database. The next section explains how to enter insurance payments.

Entering Insurance Payments in Medisoft

After an RA is received and the payment information on it is verified, the next step is to enter the payment information into the database. In Medisoft, payment information from an RA is entered in the Deposit List window (see Figure 6-7). The Deposit List window is opened by clicking Enter Deposits/Payments on the Activities menu.

The first thing you do when entering a deposit is enter the date of the deposit in the Deposit Date field. Then the New button is clicked to enter specific information about the deposit in the Deposit window (see Figure 6-8). First, the option in the Payor Type field is selected to indicate whether the payment is a patient, insurance, or capitation payment. Then the payment method, the check number, a description, the amount of the payment, and the insurance carrier are entered. After the entries are completed, the Save button is clicked. The entry then appears in the Deposit List window.

Insurance payments must be applied to specific patients, cases, dates, and procedures. To do this, the Apply button in the Deposit List window is clicked. The amount of the payment appears in the upper right corner

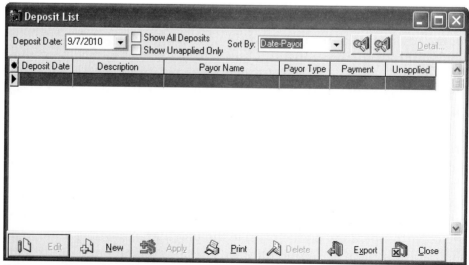

Figure 6-7 *Deposit List Window*

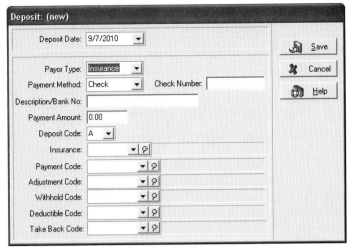

Figure 6-8 *Deposit Window*

under the heading Unapplied Amount. As you apply payments, this amount decreases until it reaches zero. To begin applying the payment, a patient's chart number is selected in the For field. The program then lists that patient's unpaid charges. Using information on the RA, the appropriate payment amounts in the Payment and Allowed columns for each procedure charge are entered and the Tab key is pressed. When you are finished entering payments for that patient, save your work by clicking the Save Payments/Adjustments button.

If the payment is for more than one patient, you can continue applying the payment by selecting the next patient in the For field. Remember to click the Save Payments/Adjustments button each time you finish working with a specific patient.

If you make an error when entering a deposit, select the deposit in the Deposit List window and click the Delete button. If the deposit has already been applied to patient accounts, the payments will also need to be deleted from the Transaction Entry window for each patient.

> **$ BILLING TIP**
>
> *Before you delete a deposit in the Deposit List window, select the deposit and click the Detail button. If the payment has already been applied, Medisoft lists the details of how it was applied. Delete the corresponding payments in the Transaction Entry window. Then delete the deposit in the Deposit List window.*

Computer Practice 6-7: *Recording Payments from an Insurance Carrier (Blue Cross and Blue Shield)*

Family Care Center received an RA from Blue Cross and Blue Shield for several patients. Enter the deposit and apply the payments using the information in Source Document 17.

1. Change the Medisoft Program Date to September 7, 2010.

2. Click Enter Deposits/Payments on the Activities menu. The Deposit List window is displayed. Verify that the date in the Deposit Date field is 9/7/2010 and that both boxes to the right of the date field (Show All Deposits and Show Unapplied Only) are unchecked.

3. Click the New button. (If a Confirm dialog box appears, indicating that you have entered a future date and asking whether you want to change the date, click the No button, and then click the New button again.)

4. The Deposit (new) window is displayed.

5. Refer to the RA in Source Document 17, and fill in the fields as indicated in the following steps. Confirm that the entry in the Deposit Date box is 9/7/2010, the date on the RA.

6. Since this is a payment from an insurance carrier, verify that the selection in the Payor Type box is Insurance.

7. Select Electronic in the Payment Method box.

8. Enter *36094251* in the EFT Tracer box.

9. The Description/Bank No. field can be left blank.

10. In the Payment Amount box, enter *575.20,* the amount shown in the Amount field on the RA.

11. Accept the default entry (A) in the Deposit Code box.

12. Select 4—Blue Cross Blue Shield from the Insurance drop-down list. When an insurance carrier is selected in the Insurance box, Medisoft automatically enters codes in the remaining fields.

13. Click the Save button to save the entry, and close the Deposit window.

14. The Deposit List box reappears, with the insurance payment appearing in the list of deposits. The payment must now be applied to the specific procedure charges to which it is related.

15. With the Blue Cross/Blue Shield payment entry highlighted, click the Apply button. The Apply Payment/Adjustments to Charges window appears. *Note:* In the list of options at the bottom of the box, make sure the first three boxes are checked (see Figure 6-9).

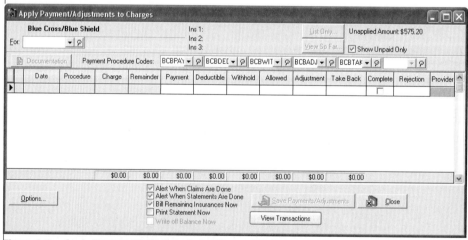

Figure 6-9 *Apply Payment/Adjustments to Charges Window*

16. Key *F* in the For box, and press Enter to select Stanley Feldman, since he is listed first on the RA. All the charge entries for Feldman that have not been paid in full are listed in the window.

17. Based on the RA, this payment is for the 93015 procedure completed on 7/28/2010. Notice that the cursor is flashing in the Payment box for this transaction.

18. Look up the amount paid to the provider on the RA. Key *260* in the Payment box, and press Tab. Medisoft automatically places a minus sign before the amount. Continue to press Tab until you get to the Allowed column.

19. Look up the allowed amount for this procedure on the RA. Enter *325* in the Allowed column, and press Tab. *Note:* In some cases, an allowed amount is already displayed in the Allowed column from a previous payment application for the same procedure. Simply key the allowed amount from the RA in place of whatever entry appears on the screen.

20. Continue to press Tab until the cursor reaches the end of the line and the amount in the Remainder column (column 4) is updated. In this case, since Blue Cross and Blue Shield pays 80 percent of the allowed amount for each procedure, the amount paid to the provider ($260) is equal to 80 percent of the allowed amount ($325).

21. Notice that the Complete box at the end of the row is checked now that the payment is applied, and that the Unapplied Amount displayed in the upper right corner of the window has been reduced from $575.20 to $315.20.

22. Since this is the only payment for Stanley Feldman on this RA, click the Save Payments/Adjustments button to save your entry.

23. An Information box appears, stating that the claim has been marked done for the primary insurance carrier. Click the OK button. The window is cleared of the current transactions and is ready for a new transaction.

24. Since Marion Johnson is next on the RA, select Marion Johnson from the For list, and apply the four Blue Cross and Blue Shield payments listed on the RA to her August 18 and August 30 charges. Remember to:

   - Make entries in the Payment column for each procedure based on the Amount Paid Provider column on the RA.

   - Make entries in the Allowed column for each procedure based on the Allowed Amount column on the RA.

   - Tab to the end of the row until the Remainder amount is updated.

   - Click the Save Payments/Adjustments button to save your work after you finish applying all four of Marion Johnson's payments.

25. Select the third patient on the RA, James Smith, in the For field, and apply the payments to his July 8 and August 17 charges in the same way. Before you click the button to save your work, notice that the Unapplied Amount area in the upper right corner of the window for the Blue Cross and Blue Shield payment is now 0.00. Click the Save Payments/Adjustments button to save your work.

26. Click the Close button to exit the Apply Payment/Adjustments to Charges window. The Unapplied column in the far right of the Deposit List window says 0.00, indicating that full amount of the payment has been applied.

Computer Practice 6-8: *Recording Payments from an Insurance Carrier (TRICARE)*

A remittance advice (RA) has been received from TRICARE for several patients. Enter the deposit, and apply the payments using Source Document 18.

1. Click the New button in the Deposit List window. (If a Confirm box appears asking whether you want to change the date, Click No, and then click the New button again.)

2. When the Deposit window appears, confirm that the entry in the Deposit Date box is 9/7/2010, the date on the RA.

3. Verify that the selection in the Payor Type box is Insurance.

4. Enter Electronic in the Payment Method box.

5. Enter the EFT number in the EFT Tracer box.

6. Enter the amount of the payment in the Payment Amount box.

7. Accept the default entry (A) in the Deposit Code box.

8. Select the insurance carrier from the Insurance drop-down list.

9. Click the Save button to save the entry and close the Deposit window.

10. The Deposit List window reappears. The insurance payment appears in the list of deposits.

11. With the TRICARE payment entry highlighted, click the Apply button.

12. Apply the payments to the appropriate charges. Remember to make entries in the Payment and Allowed columns for each payment and to tab to the end of the row to update the Remainder amount. Since TRICARE is a managed care plan, notice that the amount charged by the provider and the amount allowed by the payer are not the same. The allowed amount for each procedure is 90 percent of the amount charged. In addition, as listed on the RA, patients have already paid a $10 copay for each visit.

13. After entering the payments for each patient, click the Save Payments/Adjustments button to save your entries.

14. Click the Close button to exit the Apply Payment/Adjustments to Charges window.

$ BILLING TIP

Sometimes you may want to look up information about the services a patient received before you apply a payment. The View Transactions button in the Apply Payment/ Adjustments to Charges window can be used to view patients' transactions in the Transaction Entry window without having to exit the Apply Payment/ Adjustments to Charges window. Data in the Transaction Entry window can be viewed but not edited. When you close the window, you are returned to the Apply Payments/ Adjustments to Charges window.

Computer Practice 6-9: *Recording Payments from an Insurance Carrier (Blue Cross and Blue Shield)*

Family Care Center received an RA from Blue Cross and Blue Shield for Cedera and Lisa Lomos. Enter the deposit and apply the payments using the information in Source Document 19.

1. Confirm that the Medisoft Program Date is September 7, 2010.

2. Click the New button in the Deposit List window.

3. When the Deposit window appears, enter the information about the payment, as shown on the RA, and click the Save button.

4. Apply the payments to the appropriate charges. Remember to make entries in the Payment and Allowed columns for each payment and to tab to the end of the line. Be sure to save your work.

5. Click the Close button to exit the Apply Payment/Adjustments to Charges window.

Adjustments

As discussed earlier, the amount a physician is reimbursed for a service depends on the patient's insurance benefits and the provider's agreement with the insurance carrier. Providers establish a list of standard fees for procedures and services. Payers also develop a list of standard fees, but this payment schedule is based on a rate established in a contract with the provider. Most of the time, the amount the provider bills and the rate specified in the contract with the insurance carrier differ. The difference between the amount billed and the amount paid is an adjustment that is entered in the billing area of the practice management program, and the provider absorbs the cost.

Insurance carriers may also deny payment for some procedures. This may be because a service is not covered by the patient's insurance policy or because incomplete or incorrect information was submitted on the claim. Both denials and partial payments are entered into Medisoft as adjustments. If the provider is expected to pay for the balance of the denial or partial payment, the amount remains in the adjustment column. If the patient is responsible for the unpaid portion, the amount in the adjustment column is deleted so that the unpaid portion shifts to the remainder column, where it becomes the patient's responsibility.

Computer Practice 6-10: *Entering an Adjustment*

Family Care Center received an RA from Blue Cross and Blue Shield for two of Ellen Barmenstein's visits. Enter the deposit and apply the payments using the information in Source Document 20. Because the insurance carrier did not pay for one of the procedures on September 3, you will need to enter an adjustment.

1. Open the Deposit List window, if it is not already open.

2. Verify that the Deposit Date field displays 9/7/2010.

3. Click the New button.

4. Refer to the RA, and enter the information about the payment in the Deposit window. Then click the Save button.

5. With the payment highlighted in the Deposit List window, click the Apply button.

6. Select Barmenstein's chart number.

BILLING TIP

To move forward through the fields in the Apply Payment/Adjustments to Charges window, press Tab. To move backward, press Shift + Tab.

7. Enter the payment and the allowed amount for the charge on August 28, 2010.

8. Enter the zero payment and zero allowed amount for the first charge listed for September 3, 2010 (procedure code 99211). Notice that the RA provides a note explaining the zero payment. (The insurance plan does not cover this procedure in combination with procedure 90471.) After you enter the zero payment, the adjustment column displays –30.00.

9. Assume that the provider explained to Barmenstein, prior to the procedure, that she would be responsible for the unpaid amount. To change the responsibility for the $30 to the patient, edit the –30.00 in the adjustment column to 00.00. Tab to the end of the line.

10. The $30.00 is now displayed in the Remainder column, indicating that the patient, rather than the practice, is responsible for the noncovered procedure.

11. Enter the payments and the allowed amounts for the other two charges on the RA.

12. Save the entry, and close the Apply Payment/Adjustments to Charges window.

13. Close the Deposit List window.

✓CHECKPOINT

5. Which menu is used to select the Enter Deposits/Payments option?

6. What is the difference between the allowed amount and the amount charged by the provider?

7. If an insurance plan does not pay for a procedure, what should be entered in the Payment column in the Apply Payment/Adjustments to Charges window?

Creating Patient Statements

A **patient statement** lists the amount of money a patient owes, organized by the amount of time the money has been owed, the procedures performed, and the dates the procedures were performed. Figure 6-10 shows a sample patient statement. In earlier versions of Medisoft, statements were created from the Reports menu. Beginning with Version 9, statements are created using the Statement Management feature.

Statement Management Window

Just as the Claim Management window provides a range of options for billing insurance carriers, the Statement Management window, as illustrated

PB Family Care Center	Statement Date	Chart Number	Page
285 Stephenson Boulevard			
Stephenson, OH 60089	09/07/2010	SMIJA000	1
(614)555-0100			

Make Checks Payable To:

PB Family Care Center
285 Stephenson Boulevard
Stephenson, OH 60089
(614)555-0100

James L. Smith
17 Blacks Lane
Stephenson, OH 60089

Date of Last Payment: 9/7/2010	Amount: -70.40	Previous Balance:	8.80

Patient:	James L. Smith		Chart Number: SMIJA000		Case:	Chest pains	

Dates	Procedure	Charge	Paid by Primary	Paid By Guarantor	Adjustments	Remainder
08/17/10	99212	44.00	-35.20		0.00	8.80

Amount Due
17.60

Figure 6-10   *Sample Patient Statement*

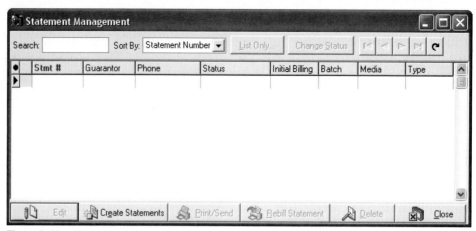

Figure 6-11   *Statement Management Window*

in Figure 6-11, offers multiple choices for billing patients. Within this window, statements are created and printed. The Statement Management window is displayed by clicking Statement Management on the Activities menu or by clicking the shortcut button on the toolbar.

Creating Patient Statements

After you create, transmit, and process insurance claims, it is time to create patient statements to inform patients of their account balance. Statements are created by clicking the Create Statements button in the Statement Management window, which displays the Create Statements window (see Figure 6-12).

In the Create Statements window, you can create statements for all transactions, or you can create only those statements that match certain criteria.

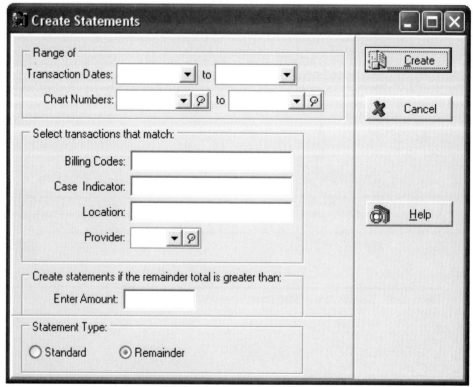

Figure 6-12   *Create Statements Window*

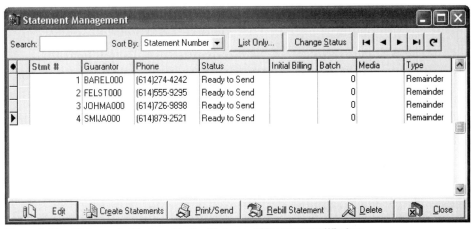

Figure 6-13 *Statements Displayed in the Statement Management Window*

Statements can be filtered by transaction dates, chart numbers, billing codes, case indicators, locations, and providers.

There is also an option to limit the creation of statements to accounts that have balances at or above a certain dollar amount. For example, a practice may have a policy that statements are not mailed to patients whose accounts have balances below $5.00.

In addition, the type of statement must be specified. Medisoft offers two options: standard and remainder. **Standard statements** show all charges regardless of whether the insurance carrier has paid on the transactions. **Remainder statements** list only those charges that are not paid in full after all insurance carrier payments have been received. Once a statement type is selected, the setting remains in effect until the other type of statement is selected.

After all selections are complete in the Create Statements window, clicking the Create button instructs the program to generate statements. The Medisoft application looks at each charge to determine whether it has been paid in full or if a balance remains. After the program determines which statements to generate, it automatically creates the statements, assigns a number, and displays a list of the statements in the Statement Management window. As shown in Figure 6-13, the status of the new statements is Ready to Send, and the default type is Remainder.

> **$ BILLING TIP**
>
> *Medisoft does not create statements for patients with zero balances. If you try to create a statement for such a patient, the following message appears: "No new statements were created." Click OK to close the dialog box that contains the message.*

Computer Practice 6-11: *Creating Statements*

Create remainder statements for all patients with outstanding balances of $5.00 or more.

1. Verify that the Medisoft Program Date is September 7, 2010.

2. Select Statement Management on the Activities menu.

3. Click the Create Statements button.

4. Enter *9/7/2010* in the second Transaction Dates box. (If a Confirm dialog box appears asking you if you want to change the date you entered, click No.)

5. Enter *5.00* in the Enter Amount box in the Create Statements If the Remainder Total Is Greater Than field, if it is not already entered.

6. Make sure that the Remainder radio button is selected. Leave all other boxes as they are.

7. Click the Create button. A message is displayed indicating the number of statements that were created.

8. Click the OK button. The Statement Management window displays the list of statements that were created.

Printing Statements

Once statements have been created, the next step is to print and mail them or to send them electronically. When the Print/Send button is clicked, the Print/Send Statements window is displayed (see Figure 6-14). This box lists options for choosing the type of statement that will be created—Paper or Electronic. Paper statements are printed and mailed by the practice. Electronic statements are sent electronically to a processing center that prints and mails them.

Once these selections are made, the OK button is clicked, and the Open Report window appears. The report selected in this window must match the type of statement selected in the Statement Type field of the Create Statements window—either Standard or Remainder. If Remainder was checked, statements will print only if one of the four Remainder Statement report formats is selected in the Open Report window. The same is true for Standard Statements.

After the report format is selected, clicking the OK button displays the Print Report Where? window, which asks whether you want to preview the report on screen, send the report directly to the printer, or export the report to a file format.

Once the Start button is clicked, the Data Selection Questions window appears (see Figure 6-15). The fields in the Data Selection Questions window are used to filter statement selections. For example, to print statements for a certain group of patients, entries are made in the Chart Number Range field. Many practices use cycle billing rather than **once-a-month billing** in which all statements are printed and mailed at once. In a **cycle billing** system, patients are divided into groups, and statement printing

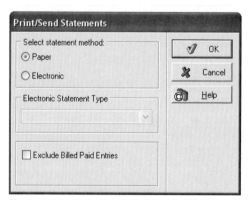

Figure 6-14   *Print/Send Statements Window*

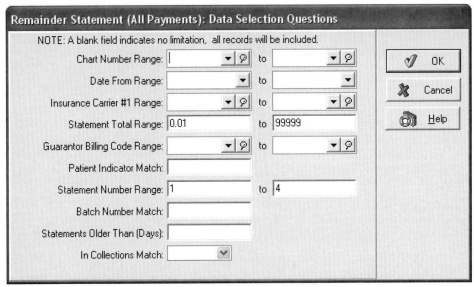

Remainder Statement (All Payments): Data Selection Questions

NOTE: A blank field indicates no limitation, all records will be included.

Chart Number Range: [ ] to [ ]

Date From Range: [ ] to [ ]

Insurance Carrier #1 Range: [ ] to [ ]

Statement Total Range: 0.01 to 99999

Guarantor Billing Code Range: [ ] to [ ]

Patient Indicator Match: [ ]

Statement Number Range: 1 to 4

Batch Number Match: [ ]

Statements Older Than (Days): [ ]

In Collections Match: [ ]

OK

Cancel

Help

Figure 6-15   *Data Selection Questions Window That Appears When Printing Remainder Statements*

and mailing is staggered throughout the month. For example, statements for guarantors whose last names begin with the letters *A* to *F* are mailed on the first of the month, those with last names that begin with *G* to *L* are mailed on the eighth of the month, and so on.

In addition to the Chart Number Range filter, a number of additional filters are available, including a filter for selecting dates, insurance carriers, account balances, and other options. Once all selections are complete, clicking the OK button sends the statements to a printer, to an electronic statement processor, or to a file, depending on the option selected earlier in the Print Report Where? window.

Computer Practice 6-12: *Printing Patient Statements*

1. Click the Print/Send button in the Statement Management window.

2. Verify that the statement method button for paper is selected. Click the OK button. The Open Report window appears.

3. Select Remainder Statement (All Payments), and click the OK button.

4. Choose to preview the report on the screen, and click the Start button.

5. Select BAREL000 in both of the Chart Number Range fields to view a patient statement for Ellen Barmenstein.

6. Enter *8/1/2010* and *9/7/2010* in the Date From Range boxes. Then click the OK button.

7. Review the patient statement.

8. Print the report after making sure that it includes only one statement.

9. Close the Preview Report window. Notice that the status of the statement in the Statement Management window is now Sent. Once a statement is printed, the status automatically changes to Sent.

10. Close the Statement Management window.

8. Which option from the Activities menu do you select to access the Statement Management functions?

9. If a patient has a zero balance, will Medisoft create a statement for that patient?

10. Which type of statement lists all charges regardless of whether a payment has been made?

11. After statements are printed, what status does the program assign to those statements?

Computer Practice 6-13: *Exiting the Program and Making a Backup Copy*

Exit the software, and make a backup copy of your work by following these steps.

1. Choose Exit from the File menu, or use the toolbar to select this option.

2. Click the Back Up Data Now button.

3. In the Destination File Path and Name box, enter the location where the backup file will be saved (if it is not already displayed). Name the new file *PBChap6.mbk.*

4. Click the Start Backup button. When the Backup Complete box appears, click OK. The Medisoft program shuts down.

CHAPTER 6 Review

DEFINE THE TERMS

Write a definition for each term: (Obj. 6-1)

1. Claim status

   _____

   _____

2. Clearinghouse

   _____

   _____

3. Cycle billing

   _____

   _____

4. EDI receiver

   _____

   _____

5. Once-a-month billing

   _____

   _____

6. Patient statement

   _____

   _____

7. Remainder statements

   _____

   _____

8. Remittance advice (RA)

   _____

   _____

9. Standard statements

   _____

   _____

10. What status does the program assign to the new claims it creates? What other status options are used by the program? (Obj. 6-2)

_____

_____

11. Can you edit claims after you create them? Why might you need to edit a claim? (Obj. 6-4)

_____

_____

12. When does the Medisoft program automatically mark claims to indicate that they were sent? (Objs. 6-2, 6-4, 6-5, 6-6)

_____

_____

13. Why would you use the option to delete a claim? (Obj. 6-6)

_____

_____

14. Where is payment information from a remittance advice (RA) first entered in Medisoft? (Obj. 6-7)

_____

_____

15. When applying payments in the Apply Payment/Adjustments to Charges window, how do you know when the full amount of the deposit has been applied? (Obj. 6-7)

_____

_____

16. What type of statement would you choose if you wanted to bill a patient for the amount due after all payments were received from insurance carriers? (Obj. 6-9)

_____

_____

17. What window is used to filter statements before they are printed? (Obj. 6-10)

_____

_____

CRITICAL ANALYSIS EXERCISES

18. List the steps you would take to create and process claims. (Obj. 6-2)

_____

_____

_____

_____

19. In the Apply Payment/Adjustments to Charges window, when does Medisoft automatically enter an adjustment? (Obj. 6-8)

_____

_____

20. List the steps you would take to create statements for all patients with account balances above $1.00. (Obj. 6-10)

_____

_____

_____

_____

ON-SCREEN REVIEW

Answer the following questions based on the results of the computer practice exercises in this chapter.

21. What procedure and date is listed on Cedera Lomos's insurance claim?

_____

22. On the printed claim for Sarina Bell, what date appears in the Signature on File field at the bottom of the claim? (_Hint:_ To view the claim again, select the claim in the Claim Management window, and click the Reprint Claim button. Select the Laser CMS (Primary) W/Form report format to view the data and form together in the preview window.)

_____

23. In the Deposit List window, enter the date **9/7/2010** in the Deposit Date box. Select the TRICARE payment dated 9/7/2010. Click the Detail button in the upper right corner of the window. Based on the information displayed, how much of the TRICARE payment was applied to Ann Peterson's account?

_____

24. How many patient statements are listed in the Statement Management window?

_____

25. What amount is displayed in the Amount Due box at the bottom of Ellen Barmenstein's patient statement?

_____

Producing Reports

WHAT YOU NEED TO KNOW

To complete this chapter, you need to know how to:

- Enter information in Medisoft.
- Navigate the Medisoft software.
- Search for information in a Medisoft database.
- Enter patient and case information.
- Record procedure charges and payments.

WHAT YOU WILL LEARN

When you finish this chapter, you will be able to complete the following objectives:

7-1. Define the terms introduced in the chapter.

7-2. Describe the steps used to print a report and export a report to a PDF file.

7-3. Print Patient Day Sheet and Procedure Day Sheet reports.

7-4. Create two types of analysis reports.

7-5. Learn about two types of aging reports.

7-6. Discuss the purpose of collection reports.

7-7. Print a Patient Ledger report.

7-8. Print a Standard Patient List report.

7-9. Access the built-in custom reports, and print various custom list reports.

7-10. Describe how to create a custom report.

KEY TERMS

Aging The classification of accounts receivable by the length of time an account is past due.

Billing/Payment Status report A report that lists the status of all transactions having a responsible insurance carrier, showing who has paid and who has not been billed.

Cash flow Movement of money from patients into a practice and to suppliers and staff out of a practice. Refers to actual cash as opposed to receivables and payables.

Insurance Aging report A report that shows an aging analysis of insurance accounts.

Insurance Collection reports Reports that are used to monitor outstanding claim balances of insurance carriers.

Patient Aging Applied Payment report Detailed report that shows an aging analysis of patient accounts.

Patient Collection report A report that is used to identify outstanding patient balances and monitor the collections process.

Patient Ledger report A report that lists the account activity for each patient for a specified time period and shows the current balance and any unpaid charges.

Payables Money owed by a practice but not yet sent to suppliers.

Practice Analysis report Detailed report that shows the practice's revenue for a period of time.

Receivables Money owed to a medical practice but not yet received from patients and insurance companies.

Medisoft Reports

The reports produced by the Medisoft program contain a variety of useful information about a medical practice and its patients. The office manager, the providers, and you, as the billing assistant, may have different informational needs for the data provided on the various reports. For example, you might use the Patient Day Sheet to verify a bank deposit, since this report shows the cash received during the day. Other reports may help the office manager track the medical practice's **cash flow,** or movement of money into and out of the practice.

$BILLING TIP

In many printed reports, Medisoft prints the Windows System Date somewhere on the report. For the purposes of these exercises, this date is not important. It is simply the date that you actually completed the exercise and does not effect the data in the report itself.

Information regarding receivables and payables, along with aging data, is also used to manage the financial aspects of a medical practice. **Receivables,** which represent money owed to a practice by its patients and insurance carriers, must be constantly tracked. Reports that show aging data classify receivables by the length of time an account is past due. An office manager could use these data to find out which patients or companies have accounts that are past due. **Payables,** or amounts due to suppliers, must be managed, too.

Some of the reports that you can print using the Medisoft program are listed below. These reports are accessed via the Reports menu (see Figure 7-1).

Day Sheets

Day Sheet reports summarize activity during a specific period. Typically, these reports are printed at the end of each day. You can use them as a backup for the day's transactions, to verify the cash on hand with the receipts listed on the report, and to analyze the revenue for the day.

The Patient Day Sheet summarizes the procedures, charges, payments, and adjustments by patient. The Procedure Day Sheet provides similar information, but it is organized by procedure codes. The Payment Day Sheet report lists the transactions for the day, or for a range of days, as well as all payments made toward those transactions. Payments are listed by the entry numbers assigned by Medisoft.

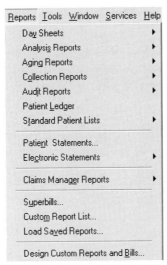

Figure 7-1 *Medisoft Reports Menu*

The first step in creating a day sheet after the option is selected on the Reports menu is to complete the Data Selection Questions window. Some version of this window is used with all Medisoft reports to select the range of data that will be included in a report. The Data Selection Questions window that is used with a Patient Day Sheet is illustrated in Figure 7-2. If any box in the Data Selection Questions window is left blank, all values are included in the report. For example, if no chart numbers are entered, all patients will be included in the report.

The Date Created Range boxes in the various Data Selection Questions windows refer to the actual date the information was entered in the computer. By default, Medisoft enters the Windows System Date in both Date Created Range boxes. In previous versions of Medisoft, it was possible to

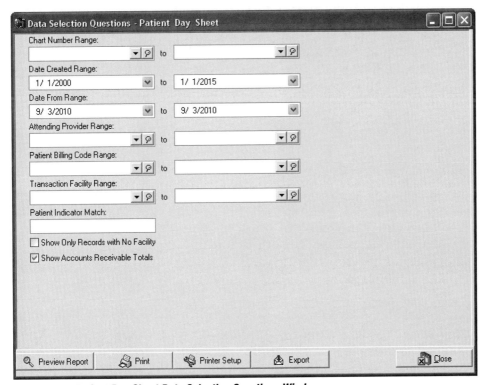

Figure 7-2 *Patient Day Sheet Data Selection Questions Window*

delete the default entries in the Date Created Range boxes and leave the boxes blank so that all values could be included in the report. In Version 14, the Date Created Range boxes cannot be left blank. Some value must be entered. Therefore, for the purposes of the exercises in this text/workbook, whenever an all-inclusive range is required for this field, always enter 1/1/2000 in the first box and 1/1/2015 in the second box. By using this broad range of dates, you can be certain that all the data you entered will be included in the report.

Computer Practice 7-1: *Printing a Patient Day Sheet*

Print a patient day sheet report for September 3, 2010, for the full range of patients.

1. Start the Medisoft program.

2. Set the program date to September 3, 2010.

3. Restore the backup file that you created at the end of Chapter 6.

4. Open the Reports menu, choose Day Sheets, and choose the Patient Day Sheet option.

5. The Data Selection Questions window appears. Leave the Chart Number Range boxes blank in order to include all patients in the report.

6. The Windows System Date—that is, the date on which you are working on this exercise—will likely appear in both Date Created Range boxes. Enter *1/1/2000* in the first Date Created Range box, and enter *1/1/2015* in the second box.

7. In the Date From Range boxes, enter *9/3/2010* for the beginning and ending dates to print a day sheet for September 3, 2010.

8. Click the box at the bottom of the window to show the accounts receivable totals at the end of the report. The Data Selection Questions window should now look like the one shown in Figure 7-2 above.

9. Click the Preview Report button.

10. After a few moments, the report (as illustrated in Figure 7-3) should appear on your screen in the preview window. (You may need to enlarge your preview window by dragging the right edge to the right to view the full width of the report.) The buttons on the toolbar at the top of the preview window let you perform various functions. If you place the cursor over a button, the name of the button is displayed. Try viewing the name of each button.

11. The zoom button currently displays "100%." Pull down the zoom menu to view other options. You can also key another percentage in the box, for example, 115, to fine-tune the percentage. View the information shown on page 1 of the report.

12. Click the Go to Next Page button (right arrow) to view each page of the report.

13. Click the Printer button to print the report.

14. Exit the preview window by clicking the X in the upper right corner of the screen.

PB Family Care Center

Patient Day Sheet

September 03, 2010
9/3/2010

Entry	Date	Document	POS	Description	Provider	Code	Modifiers	Amount
BAREL000 Barmenstein, Ellen								
221	9/3/2010	1009030000	11	OF--Established patient, minimal	1	99211		30.00
222	9/3/2010	1009030000	11	Immunization administration	1	90471		10.00
223	9/3/2010	1009030000	11	Influenza injection, older than 3 years	1	90658		12.00

Patient's Charges	Patient's Receipts	Insurance Receipts	Adjustments	Patient Balance
$52.00	$0.00	$0.00	$0.00	$43.20

Entry	Date	Document	POS	Description	Provider	Code	Modifiers	Amount
BELSA001 Bell, Sarina								
228	9/3/2010	1009030000	11	OF--Established patient, low	1	99212		44.00
229	9/3/2010	1009030000	11	Strep screen	1	87430		32.00
230	9/3/2010	1009030000	11	CBC w/diff	1	85025	90	25.00
231	9/3/2010	1009030000	11	USLife Patient Copayment	1	USLCOP		-15.00

Patient's Charges	Patient's Receipts	Insurance Receipts	Adjustments	Patient Balance
$101.00	-$15.00	$0.00	$0.00	$86.00

Entry	Date	Document	POS	Description	Provider	Code	Modifiers	Amount
JONEL000 Jones, Elizabeth								
226	9/3/2010	1009030000	11	OF--Established patient, low	1	99212		44.00
227	9/3/2010	1009030000	11	USLife Patient Copayment	1	USLCOP		-15.00

Patient's Charges	Patient's Receipts	Insurance Receipts	Adjustments	Patient Balance
$44.00	-$15.00	$0.00	$0.00	$88.00

Entry	Date	Document	POS	Description	Provider	Code	Modifiers	Amount
LOMCE000 Lomos, Cedera								
217	9/3/2010	1009030000	11	OF--New patient, moderate	1	99204		147.00

Patient's Charges	Patient's Receipts	Insurance Receipts	Adjustments	Patient Balance
$147.00	$0.00	$0.00	$0.00	$29.40

Entry	Date	Document	POS	Description	Provider	Code	Modifiers	Amount
LOMLI000 Lomos, Lisa								
218	9/3/2010	1009030000	11	Preventive new, 5-11 years	1	99383		140.00

Patient's Charges	Patient's Receipts	Insurance Receipts	Adjustments	Patient Balance
$140.00	$0.00	$0.00	$0.00	$28.00

Entry	Date	Document	POS	Description	Provider	Code	Modifiers	Amount
MITCA000 Mitchell, Caroline								
232	9/3/2010	1009030000	11	Patient payment, check	1	02		-60.00

Patient's Charges	Patient's Receipts	Insurance Receipts	Adjustments	Patient Balance
$0.00	-$60.00	$0.00	$0.00	$0.00

Entry	Date	Document	POS	Description	Provider	Code	Modifiers	Amount
PATLE000 Patterson, Leila								
219	9/3/2010	1009030000	11	OF--Established patient, low	1	99212		44.00
220	9/3/2010	1009030000	11	Cholesterol test	1	82465		21.00

Patient's Charges	Patient's Receipts	Insurance Receipts	Adjustments	Patient Balance
$65.00	$0.00	$0.00	$0.00	$65.00

Figure 7-3   *Sample Page from a Patient Day Sheet Report*

Crystal Reports Preview Window

You may have noticed that the preview window used in the exercise above was different from the preview window used in Chapter 6 to preview claims. The preview window used with the Day Sheet report in Chapter Practice 7-1 is powered by Crystal Reports software inside Medisoft. The Crystal Reports Preview window became available with Medisoft Version 12 and is used with most of the options on the Reports menu in Version 14. The preview window used earlier in Chapter 6 to preview claims is Medisoft's standard preview window. The standard preview window is still used to view claims, as well as Medisoft custom reports, which are discussed at the end of the chapter.

Although both preview windows function in the same way, the toolbar in the Crystal Reports window offers more options. The export button in the Crystal Reports preview toolbar, for example, can be used to export the report data to a variety of file types, including Adobe PDF, Microsoft Word, Microsoft Excel, and text files. You will practice exporting data in the next exercise. In the standard Medisoft preview window, the Save Report to Disk button can be used to save the report to a Medisoft Quick Report file type (*.QRP) only. Other buttons on the Crystal Reports preview toolbar (see Figure 7-4) can be used to print the report, refresh the data, jump to different sections in the report (via the Toggle Group Tree button), zoom in on the report, move from page to page, stop the loading of a report, perform a text search in the report, and access the Medisoft built-in Help feature.

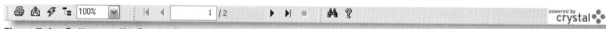

Figure 7-4 *Buttons on the Crystal Reports Preview Toolbar*

Computer Practice 7-2: *Printing a Procedure Day Sheet and Exporting the Report to a PDF File*

Print a procedure day sheet report for September 3, 2010, with the full range of procedure codes, and export the report to a PDF file.

1. Verify that the program date is September 3, 2010.

2. Select the option to print a Procedure Day Sheet.

3. In the Data Selection Questions window, leave the Procedure Code Range boxes blank in order to include all procedure codes in the report.

4. In the Date Created Range boxes, change the entries to *1/1/2000* and *1/1/2015.*

5. Enter *9/3/2010* in both of the Date From Range boxes to print a procedure day sheet for September 3, 2010.

6. Click the box at the bottom of the window to show the accounts receivable totals.

7. Click the Preview Report button to display the procedure day sheet report.

8. Review both pages of the report.

9. Click the print button to print the report.

10. Click the Export Report button to export the report to a PDF file in order to store it for future use.

11. When the Export dialog box appears, click the OK button to accept the default format (Acrobat format, PDF) and the default destination (Disk File), as shown in Figure 7-5.

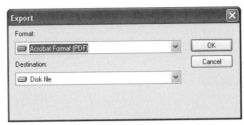

Figure 7-5 *Export Dialog Box*

12. In the next dialog box, accept the default print range to print all pages.

13. When prompted for a file name, save the file in the same folder where your Medisoft backup files are stored (for example, under My Documents, in a folder named PB7e), or ask your instructor where to save the file. Name the file *Exercise 7-2.* Click Save.

14. Exit the preview window.

Analysis Reports

Several reports can be prepared with the Medisoft program that are useful in analyzing a medical practice's financial activity. These reports include the Billing/Payment Status report and the Practice Analysis report. Each report provides a different perspective of the financial data stored in the patient accounting system.

Billing/Payment Status Report

The **Billing/Payment Status report** is an excellent practice management tool. It lists the status of all transactions having a responsible insurance carrier, showing who has paid and who has not been billed (see Figure 7-6 on page 146). This information is helpful in determining whether billing charges can be applied to a patient balance.

The report is sorted by Chart Number and then Case. Every chart number listed shows a patient balance and whether there have been any unapplied payments or unapplied adjustments.

Practice Analysis Report

The **Practice Analysis report** shows the total revenue for each procedure performed during a specific period (such as week, month, or year). The summary section of the report includes information such as total procedure charges, total insurance payments, total patient payments, and net effect on accounts receivable (see Figure 7-7 on page 147). This report is useful in analyzing which procedures generated the most revenue. Subsequently, the report can be used to perform a profitability analysis and may be helpful to an accountant who is preparing financial statements for the medical practice.

Billing Payment Status
1/1/2010 to 9/7/2010

Date	Document	Procedure	Amount	Policy 1	Policy 2	Policy 3	Guarantor	Adjustments	Balance
BAREL000	Ellen Barmenstein	(614)274-4242							
Case 1			1: Blue Cross/Blue Shield (614)241-9000						
8/28/2010	0508290000	99212	44.00	-35.20*	0.00*	0.00*	9/7/2010	0.00*	8.80
								Subtotal:	8.80
							Unapplied Payments and Adjustments:		0.00
								Case Balance:	8.80
Case 29			1: Blue Cross/Blue Shield (614)241-9000						
9/3/2010	1009030000	99211	30.00	0.00*	0.00*	0.00*	9/7/2010	0.00*	30.00
9/3/2010	1009030000	90471	10.00	-8.00*	0.00*	0.00*	9/7/2010	0.00*	2.00
9/3/2010	1009030000	90658	12.00	-9.60*	0.00*	0.00*	9/7/2010	0.00*	2.40
								Subtotal:	34.40
							Unapplied Payments and Adjustments:		0.00
								Case Balance:	34.40
								Patient Balance:	43.20
BELHE000	Herbert Bell	(614)241-6124							
Case 2			1: U.S. Life (800)921-6320						
8/30/2010	1108290000	93015	325.00	Not Billed	0.00*	0.00*	Not Billed	0.00*	325.00
8/30/2010	1108290000	99212	44.00	Not Billed	0.00*	0.00*	-15.00	0.00*	29.00
								Subtotal:	354.00
							Unapplied Payments and Adjustments:		0.00
								Case Balance:	354.00
								Patient Balance:	354.00
BELSA000	Samuel Bell	(614)241-6124							
Case 3			1: U.S. Life (800)921-6320						
6/29/2010	0506290000	99213	60.00	Not Billed	0.00*	0.00*	-15.00	0.00*	45.00
								Subtotal:	45.00
							Unapplied Payments and Adjustments:		0.00
								Case Balance:	45.00
Case 4			1: U.S. Life (800)921-6320						
7/15/2010	0507150000	99212	39.60	Not Billed	0.00*	0.00*	-15.00	0.00*	24.60

* indicates that this payment is complete

A date in the payment columns indicates the billing date

Figure 7-6 *Sample Page from a Billing/Payment Status Report*

		PB Family Care Center					
		Practice Analysis					
		From 9/1/2010 to 9/30/2010					
Code	Modifiers	Description	Amount	Units	Average	Costs	Net
02		Patient payment, check	-60.00	1	-60.00	0.00	-60.00
82465		Cholesterol test	21.00	1	21.00	0.00	21.00
85025	90	CBC w/diff	25.00	1	25.00	0.00	25.00
87430		Strep screen	32.00	1	32.00	0.00	32.00
90471		Immunization administration	10.00	1	10.00	0.00	10.00
90658		Influenza injection, older than 3 ye:	12.00	1	12.00	0.00	12.00
99204		OF--New patient, moderate	147.00	1	147.00	0.00	147.00
99211		OF--Established patient, minimal	30.00	1	30.00	0.00	30.00
99212		OF--Established patient, low	176.00	4	44.00	0.00	176.00
99383		Preventive new, 5-11 years	140.00	1	140.00	0.00	140.00
BCBPAY		Blue Cross Blue Shield Payment	-857.60	13	-65.97	0.00	-857.60
TRIADJ		Tricare Adjustment	-26.70	5	-5.34	0.00	-26.70
TRICOP		Tricare Patient Copayment	-10.00	1	-10.00	0.00	-10.00
TRIPAY		Tricare Payment	-200.30	5	-40.06	0.00	-200.30
USLCOP		USLife Patient Copayment	-30.00	2	-15.00	0.00	-30.00

Figure 7-7 *Sample Page from a Practice Analysis Report*

Computer Practice 7-3: *Printing a Practice Analysis Report*

Print a practice analysis report for September 2010.

1. Set the program date to September 30, 2010.

2. Select the option to print a Practice Analysis report.

3. In the Data Selection Questions window, leave the Procedure Code Range boxes blank to include all procedure codes in the report.

4. Change the entries in the Date Created Range boxes to *1/1/2000* and *1/1/2015.*

5. **Enter** *9/1/2010* in the first Date From Range field and *9/30/2010* in the second Date From Range field.

6. Click the box at the bottom of the window to show the accounts receivable totals.

7. Click the Preview Report button.

8. Review the information provided. Notice that there are two pages. Click the print button to print the report, or click the export button to save the report to a PDF file.

9. Exit the preview window.

Aging Reports

Aging is the classification of accounts receivables by the amount of time they are past due. A **Patient Aging Applied Payment report,** for example, shows the ages of all outstanding patient charges. The report classifies charges using four aging categories: Current (0–30 days), 31–60 days, 61–90 days, and 91 days or older. See the sample page from a Patient Aging Applied Payment report in Figure 7-8. This report is an important tool in collections as it can be used to easily identify patients whose accounts are past due.

PB Family Care Center

Patient Aging Applied Payment

by Date From
From January 01, 2010 to September 30, 2010

Chart # Name	Birthdate	Current 0 - 30	Past 31 - 60	Past 61 - 90	Past 91 +	Total Balance
BAREL000 Barmenstein, Ellen Last Pmt: -52.80 On: 9/7/2010	10/16/1982 (614)274-4242	34.40	8.80	0.00	0.00	43.20
BELHE000 Bell, Herbert Last Pmt: -15.00 On: 8/30/2010	3/31/1970 (614)241-6124	0.00	354.00	0.00	0.00	354.00
BELSA000 Bell, Samuel Last Pmt: -15.00 On: 7/15/2010	7/3/1996 (614)241-6124	0.00	0.00	24.60	45.00	69.60
BELSA001 Bell, Sarina Last Pmt: -15.00 On: 9/3/2010	1/21/1999 (614)241-6124	86.00	0.00	0.00	0.00	86.00
BRORA000 Brown, Rachel Last Pmt: -15.00 On: 8/21/2010	6/14/1972 (614)721-0044	0.00	50.00	0.00	0.00	50.00
FELST000 Feldman, Stanley Last Pmt: -260.00 On: 9/7/2010	1/30/1959 (614)555-9295	0.00	369.00	65.00	0.00	434.00
JOHMA000 Johnson, Marion Last Pmt: -244.80 On: 9/7/2010	10/15/1956 (614)726-9898	0.00	61.20	57.00	0.00	118.20
JONEL000 Jones, Elizabeth Last Pmt: -15.00 On: 9/3/2010	8/26/1974 (614)321-5555	29.00	59.00	0.00	0.00	88.00
LOMCE000 Lomos, Cedera Last Pmt: -117.60 On: 9/7/2010	5/21/1957 (614)221-0202	29.40	0.00	0.00	0.00	29.40
LOMLI000 Lomos, Lisa Last Pmt: -112.00 On: 9/7/2010	6/3/2004 (614)221-0202	28.00	0.00	0.00	0.00	28.00
MITHE000 Mitchell, Herbert Last Pmt: 0.00 On:	10/8/1934 (614)861-0909	0.00	60.00	0.00	0.00	60.00
PATLE000 Patterson, Leila Last Pmt: 0.00 On:	2/14/1949 (614)626-2099	65.00	0.00	0.00	0.00	65.00
PETPE000 Peterson, Peter Last Pmt: -10.00 On: 6/12/2010	8/8/1958 (614)555-2929	0.00	0.00	0.00	149.00	149.00
ROSPA000 Ross, Paula Last Pmt: -15.00 On: 6/19/2010	4/5/1986 (614)	0.00	0.00	0.00	70.00	70.00
SAMCA000 Sampson, Caroline Last Pmt: -15.00 On: 8/5/2010	1/26/1961 (614)836-4244	0.00	29.00	0.00	0.00	29.00
SAMHA000 Sampson, Hal Last Pmt: -15.00 On: 7/8/2010	4/30/1963 (614)836-4244	0.00	0.00	29.00	0.00	29.00

Figure 7-8 *Sample Page from a Patient Aging Applied Payment Report*

PB Family Care Center
Primary Insurance Aging
September 30, 2010

Date of Service	Procedure	- Past - 0 to 30	- Past - 31 to 60	- Past - 61 to 90	- Past - 91 to 120	- Past - 121 +	Total Balance
U.S. Life (10)							**(800)921-6320**
BELSA001 Sarina Bell			SS: 989-00-9938				
Birthdate: 1/21/1999		Policy: 50632			Group: 6209		
Claim: 54	Initial Billing Date: 9/3/2010		Last Billing Date: 9/3/2010				
9/3/2010	99212	$44.00	$0.00	$0.00	$0.00	$0.00	$44.00
9/3/2010	87430	$32.00	$0.00	$0.00	$0.00	$0.00	$32.00
9/3/2010	85025	$25.00	$0.00	$0.00	$0.00	$0.00	$25.00
		$101.00	$0.00	$0.00	$0.00	$0.00	$101.00
Insurance Totals:		$101.00	$0.00	$0.00	$0.00	$0.00	$101.00
Report Aging Totals:		$101.00	$0.00	$0.00	$0.00	$0.00	$101.00
Percent of Aging Total:		100.00%	0.00%	0.00%	0.00%	0.00%	100.00%

Figure 7-9 *Sample Page from a Primary Insurance Aging Report*

An **Insurance Aging report** is an excellent tool for tracking claims filed with insurance carriers. There are three insurance aging reports: Primary Insurance Aging, Secondary Insurance Aging, and Tertiary Insurance Aging. These reports provide aging information similar to the Patient Aging report. Instead of patients, however, the reports show each insurance carrier and its outstanding balance status (see Figure 7-9).

Collection Reports

Medisoft provides a number of collection reports that can be used to locate overdue patient or insurance accounts.

Patient Collection Report

The **Patient Collection report** makes it easy to identify outstanding balances, helping you manage your patient collections. The report draws information from the Statement Management area of the program and includes information such as chart number, patient name, telephone number, Statement Number, Initial Bill Date, Last Bill Date, Last Patient Payment Date, and Last Patient Payment Amount. A sample Patient Collection report is illustrated in Figure 7-10 on page 150.

```
                              PB Family Care Center
                              Patient Collection
                              September 30, 2010

       Statement  Initial Bill  Last Bill  Last Patient  Last Patient  Submission  Statement  Statement
       Number     Date          Date       Pay Date      Pay Amount    Count       Type       Total

BAREL000- Barmenstein, Ellen          Phone: (614)274-4242
           1     9/7/2010     9/7/2010                                      1      Remainder    $43.20
                                                                                                $43.20


                                                                          Report Total:        $43.20
```

Figure 7-10   *Sample Page from a Patient Collection Report*

Insurance Collection Reports

The Insurance Collection reports are similar to the Patient Collection reports, except that the listings are for insurance carriers instead of patients. The **Insurance Collection reports** are used to monitor outstanding claim balances. They are based on information in the Claim Management area of the program and provide details such as the Claim number, Chart number, and Primary (Secondary, Tertiary) Bill Date for each payer. Figure 7-11 shows a sample Primary Insurance Collection report.

The selections for the report can be filtered by Chart Number Range, Date Created Range, Initial Billing Date 1 Range (or Date 2 or 3 for secondary and tertiary claims), and Claim Status 1 Match (or Status 2 or 3 for secondary and tertiary claims).

Computer Practice 7-4: *Printing a Primary Insurance Collection Report*

Print a Primary Insurance Collection report as of September 30, 2010.

1. Verify that the program date is September 30, 2010.

2. Select the option to print a Primary Insurance Collection report.

3. Leave the default entries in the Data Selection Questions window as they are. Notice that, for this report, the program includes the expanded date range (1/1/1900–12/31/2050) in both date range fields by default to include all the data in the database for these fields. Click the Preview Report button.

4. Review the information provided. Do not print this report unless instructed otherwise.

5. Exit the preview window.

```
                            PB Family Care Center
                      Primary Insurance Collection
                            September 03, 2010


                      Primary                         Submission
Claim      Chart      Bill Date   Batch  Date Created  Count           Claim Total

1 - Medicare                                     (215)599-0205
40         WONJO000               0      7/29/2010     0                  1,030.00

                                                        Totals:           1,030.00


10 - U.S. Life                                   (800)921-6320
54         BELSA001   9/3/2010    3      9/3/2010       1                   101.00
55         JONEL000              0      9/3/2010       0                    44.00

                                                        Totals:             145.00


13 - Oxford                                      (614)555-0014
58         PATLE000              0      9/3/2010       0                    65.00

                                                        Totals:              65.00


3 - TRICARE                                      (614)241-8080
30         PETPE000              0      6/14/2010      0                   159.00

                                                        Totals:             159.00


4 - Blue Cross/Blue Shield                       (614)241-9000
31         MITCA000             0      6/16/2010      0                    60.00

                                                        Totals:              60.00

                                                   Report Total:        $1,459.00
```

Figure 7-11   *Sample Page from a Primary Insurance Collection Report*

Patient Ledgers

The **Patient Ledger report** lets you view the account activity for each patient (see Figure 7-12 on page 152). The ledger includes the procedure charges, payments, and adjustments for all patients or for selected patients. It also shows the current balance and any unpaid charges.

PB Family Care Center

Patient Account Ledger

As of 9/30/2010

Entry	Date	POS	Description	Procedure	Document	Provider	Amount
BAREL000	**Ellen Barmenstein**				(614)274-4242		
	Last Payment: -52.80		On: 9/7/2010				
86	8/28/2010	11		99212	0508290000	1	44.00
252	9/7/2010		#3574896 Blue Cross/Blue Shie	BCBPAY	0508290000	1	-35.20
221	9/3/2010	11		99211	1009030000	1	30.00
222	9/3/2010	11		90471	1009030000	1	10.00
223	9/3/2010	11		90658	1009030000	1	12.00
253	9/7/2010		#3574896 Blue Cross/Blue Shie	BCBPAY	1009030000	1	0.00
254	9/7/2010		#3574896 Blue Cross/Blue Shie	BCBPAY	1009030000	1	-8.00
255	9/7/2010		#3574896 Blue Cross/Blue Shie	BCBPAY	1009030000	1	-9.60
	Patient Totals						**43.20**
BELHE000	**Herbert Bell**				(614)241-6124		
	Last Payment: -15.00		On: 8/30/2010				
198	8/30/2010	11		99212	1108290000	1	44.00
199	8/30/2010	11		93015	1108290000	1	325.00
200	8/30/2010	11		USLCOP	1108290000	1	-15.00
	Patient Totals						**354.00**
BELSA000	**Samuel Bell**				(614)241-6124		
	Last Payment: -15.00		On: 7/15/2010				
171	6/29/2010	11		USLCOP	0407190000	1	-15.00
59	6/29/2010	11		99213	0506290000	1	60.00
167	7/15/2010	11		USLCOP	0407190000	1	-15.00
96	7/15/2010	11		99212	0507150000	1	39.60
	Patient Totals						**69.60**
BELSA001	**Sarina Bell**				(614)241-6124		
	Last Payment: -15.00		On: 9/3/2010				
228	9/3/2010	11		99212	1009030000	1	44.00
229	9/3/2010	11		87430	1009030000	1	32.00
230	9/3/2010	11		85025	1009030000	1	25.00
231	9/3/2010	11		USLCOP	1009030000	1	-15.00
	Patient Totals						**86.00**
BRORA000	**Rachel Brown**				(614)721-0044		
	Last Payment: -15.00		On: 8/21/2010				
169	8/21/2010	11		USLCOP	0407190000	1	-15.00
99	8/21/2010	11		99211	0508220000	1	30.00
100	8/21/2010	11		83718	0508220000	1	35.00
	Patient Totals						**50.00**
FELST000	**Stanley Feldman**				(614)555-9295		
	Last Payment: -260.00		On: 9/7/2010				

Figure 7-12 *Sample Page from a Patient Ledger Report*

Computer Practice 7-5: *Printing Patient Ledgers*

Print a patient ledger for all patients as of September 30, 2010.

1. Verify that the program date is September 30, 2010.

2. Open the Reports menu, and choose the Patient Ledger option.

3. The program displays the Data Selection Questions window (see Figure 7-13). (The default setting for the second Date From Range box will vary because it displays the computer's system date.) As with the Data Selection Questions windows for other reports, the options in this window are used to filter the data for the report. For example, you could print a Patient Ledger report for only one patient by entering that patient's chart number in both Chart Number Range boxes. Or you could print a report for a specific time period, such as the month of July, by entering specific dates in the Date From Range boxes. If a selection box is left blank, all values for that box are included in the report.

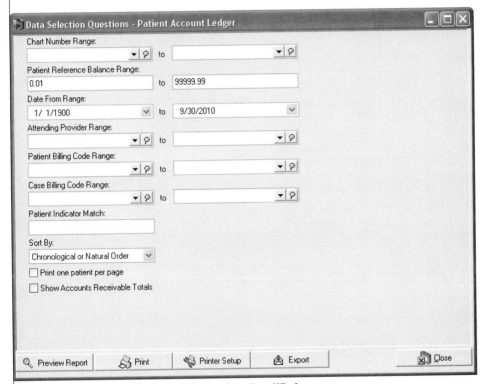

Figure 7-13 *Patient Ledger Data Selection Questions Window*

4. In this case, to print a patient ledger for all patients as of September 30, 2010, leave the Chart Number Range boxes blank. In the Date From Range boxes, leave the first date as it is (the program lists the 1/1/1900 date to include all the data in the database) and in the second Date From Range box, enter *9/30/2010.*

5. At the bottom of the window, click the box to show the accounts receivable totals. However, do *not* click the box to print one patient per page.

6. Click the Preview Report button.

7. Zoom in on the report (pages 1–4) as necessary, and review the information shown for the Family Care Center's patients.

8. Print the report, or export it to a PDF file, and then exit the preview window.

Standard Patient Lists

On the Reports menu, Medisoft includes several convenient reports for identifying patients by diagnosis, procedure, or insurance carrier. These reports are accessed via the Standard Patient Lists option (see Figure 7-14).

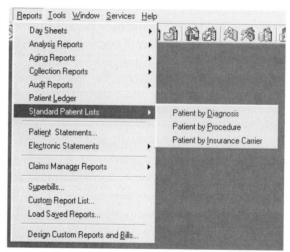

Figure 7-14 *Standard Patient Lists Option*

The Patient by Diagnosis report lists patients by diagnosis code. It also includes their chart numbers, patient names, ages, and attending providers; the facilities; and the dates of their last visits (see Figure 7-15). The Patient by Procedure report lists patients by procedure code and includes information such as chart numbers, patient names and ages, and dates of their last visits. The Patient by Insurance Carrier report lists patients, first sorted by their providers or the facility and then sorted by their insurance carriers.

Custom Reports

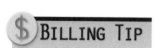

Additional custom reports and bills can be created and added to the list using the Design Custom Reports and Bills option on the Reports menu.

Medisoft stores a number of custom reports that were created using the Medisoft Report Designer. These reports come with the program and include:

- Lists of addresses, billing codes, EDI receivers, patients, patient recalls, procedure codes, providers, and referring providers
- The CMS-1500 claim forms in a variety of printer formats
- Patient statements and walkout receipts
- Superbills (encounter forms)

PB Family Care Center
Patient By Diagnosis
September 07, 2010

Diagnosis Pointer	Chart	Patient Name	Age	Attending Provider	Facility	Date of Last Visit
Diagnosis: 034.0 - Strep sore throat						
1	BELSA001	Bell, Sarina	11	1		9/3/2010
		Diagnosis: Strep sore throat Patient Count: 1				
Diagnosis: 272.0 - Hypercholesterolemia						
1	PATLE000	Patterson, Leila	61	1		9/3/2010
		Diagnosis: Hypercholesterolemia Patient Count: 1				
Diagnosis: 401.9 - Essential hypertension						
1	SAMHA000	Sampson, Hal	47	1		8/25/2010
		Diagnosis: Essential hypertension Patient Count: 1				
Diagnosis: 461.9 - Acute sinusitis						
1	SUAFE000	Suarez, Felix	58	1		9/3/2010
		Diagnosis: Acute sinusitis Patient Count: 1				
Diagnosis: 473.9 - Sinusitis - chronic						
1	LOMCE000	Lomos, Cedera	53	1		9/3/2010
		Diagnosis: Sinusitis - chronic Patient Count: 1				
Diagnosis: 490 - Bronchitis, unqualified						
1	BELSA000	Bell, Samuel	14	1		6/29/2010
		Diagnosis: Bronchitis, unqualified Patient Count: 1				
Diagnosis: 726.10 - Bursitis - shoulder						
1	WONLI000	Wong, Li Yu	72	1		8/19/2010
		Diagnosis: Bursitis - shoulder Patient Count: 1				
Diagnosis: 786.50 - Pain - chest						
1	SMIJA000	Smith, James L	31	1		8/17/2010
		Diagnosis: Pain - chest Patient Count: 1				
Diagnosis: 848.9 - Sprain or strain (no site)						
1	TANHI000	Tanaka, Hiro	10	1		9/3/2010
		Diagnosis: Sprain or strain (no site) Patient Count: 1				
Diagnosis: 870.0 - Laceration of skin or eyelid						
1	SAMCA000	Sampson, Caroline	49	1		8/5/2010
		Diagnosis: Laceration of skin or eyelid Patient Count: 1				
Diagnosis: 879.8 - Open wounds						
1	WARWI000	Ward, Winston	25	1		8/28/2010

Figure 7-15   *Sample Page from a Patient by Diagnosis Report*

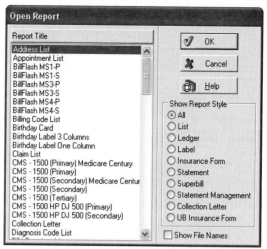

Figure 7-16 *Open Report Window with All Reports Displayed*

To access the custom reports in Medisoft, the Custom Report List option is selected on the Reports menu. The Open Report window is displayed, with a long list of reports arranged in alphabetical order (see Figure 7-16). To print a custom report, the title of the report is selected, and then the OK button is clicked.

As seen in Figure 7-16, the Open Report window contains ten radio buttons that are used to control the list of reports displayed in the window. When the All radio button is clicked, all types of custom reports are listed in the dialog box. However, when one of the other radio buttons is clicked, only reports of that style are listed. For example, if the Insurance Form radio button is clicked, only reports that are insurance forms are listed in the window.

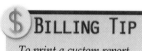

$ BILLING TIP

To print a custom report from the Open Report window, double-click the report title.

List Reports

You can use the List radio button in the Open Reports window to display only the reports that are lists. Medisoft stores most of the data for a medical practice in various databases. The data from the database can be printed as lists—procedure lists, diagnosis lists, patient lists, insurance carrier lists, and so on—by selecting the appropriate report in the Open Reports window.

Computer Practice 7-6: *Viewing Two Custom List Reports*

View the Procedure Code List report and the Patient List report.

1. Open the Reports menu, and choose Custom Report List.

2. Scroll through the list to see the full set of custom reports.

3. Click the List radio button in the Open Report window to show only the list reports (see Figure 7-17).

4. Select the Procedure Code List, and click the OK button.

5. Choose to preview the list on the screen, and click the Start button.

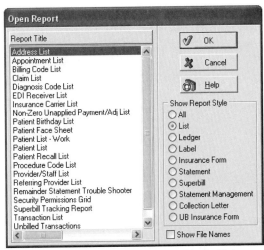

Figure 7-17 **Open Report Window with the List Reports Displayed**

6. Leave the code range boxes blank in the Data Selection Questions window to list all procedure codes. Click the OK button.

7. Review the procedures shown in the report. Note that the preview window used to display the List reports is the standard Medisoft preview window rather than the Crystal Reports preview window. Close the preview window.

8. Follow the same steps to display a patient list of all patients in the preview window. Click the print button to print the Patient List report.

9. Close the preview window.

10. Display any of the other List reports that interest you.

Designing Custom Reports and Bills

You can generate numerous custom reports in Medisoft using the Custom Report List option. However, you may want to customize a report to meet a particular need. For example, you could design a special report to be sent to an insurance carrier. In these instances, you can use the Medisoft Report Designer to modify an existing report or to create a completely new one (see Figure 7-18 on page 158). The Report Designer is a powerful tool that provides all the features you need to prepare a new report layout.

Although this text does not cover the Report Designer, you can explore this option on your own. To access the Report Designer, choose the Design Custom Reports and Bills option from the Reports menu. Remember that you can use the help feature to learn more about the Report Designer if you have questions.

Figure 7-18 *Main Window of the Medisoft Report Designer*

✓CHECKPOINT

1. Which report lists each patient account and identifies the amount of time each account has been past due?

2. Which report shows the total revenue for each procedure?

3. Which report creates a list of all procedure codes in the database?

4. Which report includes information organized by patient and is typically printed at the end of each day?

Computer Practice 7-7: *Exiting the Program and Making a Backup Copy*

Exit the software, and make a backup copy of your work by following these steps.

1. Choose Exit from the File menu, or use the toolbar to select this option.

2. Click the Back Up Data Now button.

3. In the Destination File Path and Name box, enter the location where the backup file will be saved (if it is not already displayed). Name the new file *PBChap7.mbk.*

4. Click the Start Backup button. When the Backup Complete box appears, click OK. The Medisoft program shuts down.

CHAPTER 7 Review

DEFINE THE TERMS

Write a definition for each term: (Obj. 7-1)

1. Aging

   _____

   _____

2. Billing/Payment Status report

   _____

   _____

3. Cash flow

   _____

   _____

4. Insurance Aging report

   _____

   _____

5. Insurance Collection reports

   _____

   _____

6. Patient Aging Applied Payment report

   _____

   _____

7. Patient Collection report

   _____

   _____

8. Patient Ledger report

   _____

   _____

9. Payables

   _____

   _____

10. Practice Analysis report

_____

_____

11. Receivables

_____

_____

CHECK YOUR UNDERSTANDING

12. Does the Medisoft program let you set up filters to print only selected information on a report? Explain. (Obj. 7-2)

_____

_____

_____

13. Describe how you can use the toolbar buttons in the Crystal Reports preview window to review the information in a report. (Obj. 7-2)

_____

_____

_____

14. How do the Patient and Procedure Day Sheet reports differ from one another? (Obj. 7-3)

_____

_____

_____

15. Describe how the Billing/Payment Status report can be used. (Obj. 7-4)

_____

_____

_____

16. If you were asked to print a report for all patients with outstanding balances, including the length of time each account has been unpaid, what report would you print? (Obj. 7-5)

_____

_____

_____

17. What information is included in the Patient Collection report? (Obj. 7-6)

_____

_____

_____

18. What information is included in the Patient Ledger report? (Obj. 7-7)

_____

_____

_____

19. What are the three types of Standard Patient List reports? (Obj. 7-8)

_____

_____

_____

20. Describe the type of custom list reports available in Medisoft. (Obj. 7-9)

_____

_____

_____

21. List several reasons why you might need to use the Medisoft Report Designer to customize a report. (Obj. 7-10)

_____

_____

_____

CRITICAL ANALYSIS EXERCISE

22. Why is the information on a Patient Aging Applied Payment report or a Primary Insurance Aging report so valuable in monitoring accounts receivable data? (Obj. 7-5)

_____

_____

_____

_____

Answer the following questions based on the results of the computer practice exercises in this chapter.

23. Which patients on the Patient Day Sheet report for September 3, 2010, have zero balances?

    _____

24. In the Procedure Day Sheet report for September 3, 2010, how many procedures are listed for September 3, 2010, alone? What is the balance of the charges for those procedures?

    _____

25. On page 2 of the Practice Analysis report for the month of September 2010, what is reported as the net effect on accounts receivable?

    _____

26. At the end of the Patient Account Ledger created for all patients as of September 30, 2010, what amount is reported as the ledger totals?

    _____

27. Which patients do not have phone numbers in the Patient List report for the Family Care Center?

    _____

Family Care Center: A Patient Billing Simulation

Now that you have completed the tutorial, you are ready to begin the patient billing simulation using the Medisoft program. As the new billing assistant for the Family Care Center, your job is to process the patient billing for the medical practice. The simulation takes place from Monday, November 1, 2010, through Friday, November 5, 2010. Tuesday, November 2, is Election Day, and the office is closed.

As you complete the simulation, you may notice that the volume of work is not the same as you would expect in an actual medical practice. However, the tasks you perform are similar to those a billing assistant would perform on a daily basis.

Before you begin, review the Office Procedures Manual section shown on pages 163 through 165 below. Then, refer to the step-by-step instructions for the individual days that follow on pages 165–171 to complete the simulation. If you need assistance using the software, refer to the previous chapters or use the Help information built into the software.

Office Procedures Manual

Review the office procedures for the Family Care Center. Some of these tasks are already completed for you, but in an actual office, you would perform each of these duties.

Daily Tasks Before Patients Arrive

- Assist receptionist in completing an encounter form for each patient with a scheduled appointment. Fill in the patient's name, address, and chart number and the date.

- Gather the materials for the day: the Medisoft data file and any encounter forms or receipts (cash or checks) from the previous day. The receptionist keeps the receipts in a locked drawer overnight.

- Prepare a change fund for the receptionist.

- Turn on the computer, and start Medisoft.

Morning Tasks

Each morning, you must enter the transactions and payments from the previous afternoon and then prepare a bank deposit slip. Deposits are usually made at noon.

- Enter the transaction data from the previous afternoon.
- If necessary, update any patient accounts.
- Open the mail, and record each check received. Enter the payment amount and the check number. Indicate whether the payment is from an insurer or a patient. Apply the payments to patient accounts.
- Review electronic funds transfers, and enter the payment information in Medisoft.
- Prepare a bank deposit slip for the checks received in the mail and for receipts on hand from the previous day.
- Print a patient day sheet for the previous day.
- Give the day sheets to the office manager, and take the deposit to the bank.

Afternoon Tasks

During the afternoon, your primary task is to enter the patient information, charges, and payments for patients who had morning appointments. Other tasks include transmitting claims for the previous day's transactions.

- Create and send insurance claims for the previous day's visits.
- Gather the Patient Information Forms for the new patients who had morning appointments, and enter this information into the system.
- Update any information for established patients.
- Using the encounter forms provided by the receptionist, enter the data for patients seen in the morning.
- Time permitting, enter the transactions for the afternoon appointments.
- Back up the patient billing data.

Other Tasks During the Day

- Respond to calls from patients about their accounts.
- Relieve the receptionist when needed.
- Make collection calls to patients and insurers.
- Call insurers about managed-care cases as needed.
- Fill out (or print) special forms for disability and so forth.

Weekly Tasks

- On Friday, print a Patient Aging Applied Payment report, and consult with the office manager regarding any overdue accounts. If necessary, contact patients concerning past due account balances. Write off bad debts after consulting with the office manager.

(Typically, these are for charges more than a year old where there is no chance of collecting from the patient or insurer.)

- On Friday afternoons, prepare the appropriate patient remainder statements:

  First Friday: Patients A-L
  Third Friday: Patients M-Z

- Print a Practice Analysis report.

Monday, November 1, 2010

1. Remove Source Documents 21 through 30 on pages 225–243. Review the information provided on the source documents before entering data.

2. Start the Medisoft program, and restore the backup file that you created at the end of Chapter 7.

3. Set the program date to October 29, 2010. The patient transactions from Friday afternoon, October 29, have not been recorded yet.

4. Record the transactions from last Friday following the instructions below and using the information provided on Source Documents 21–24. Use the Enter Transactions option to record the procedure charges and patient payments. Print a walkout receipt for each patient who makes a payment.

   - Use the encounter form for Janine Bell (Source Document 21) to record the procedure charge and payment.

     First you will need to create a new case. Remember to enter a description for the case based on the encounter form and to select Herbert Bell as Guarantor in the Personal tab. In addition, Janine is married but not employed. Remember to enter the diagnosis in the Diagnosis tab. When completing the Policy 1 tab, you need to know that Janine is covered by her husband's policy from U.S. Life (Policy # 50632, Group # 6209, $15 copayment). Dr. Yan accepts assignment from U.S. Life, which pays 100 percent of covered services (Box A through Box H).

     Enter the transactions, apply the payment, and print a walkout receipt.

   - Enter the information to record the procedure charge and payment for Felix Suarez (Source Document 22).

     Create a new case for this office visit. You will need to review an earlier case to get the necessary policy information, or you can copy the existing case and then change the description and diagnosis.

     Enter the transaction, apply the payment, and print a walkout receipt.

   - Record the procedure charge and payment from Sarah Fitzwilliams's encounter form (Source Document 23).

To begin, create a new case. Sarah is single and is a full-time student covered by her father's TRICARE insurance (Policy # 457091, Group # 3265, $10 copayment). Dr. Yan accepts assignment from TRICARE, which pays 100 percent of covered services (Box A through Box H).

Print a walkout receipt after entering the procedure and payment information.

- Enter the information from the encounter form for Marion Johnson (Source Document 24). Use the existing case but add an additional diagnosis.

5. Print a patient day sheet for Friday, October 29, 2010. Enter the dates *1/1/2000* and *1/1/2015* in the Date Created Range boxes, and enter *10/29/2010* in both Date From Range boxes. Be sure to check the box to show accounts receivable data at the end of the report.

6. Refer to the report to verify that you have entered the information correctly. The total charges should be $281.00, and the receipts on hand should be $−40.00. If the amounts match, continue with the next step. Otherwise, find your error, correct it, and print updated reports. After verifying the amounts, you would complete a bank deposit slip and take the deposit to the bank.

7. Create insurance claims for the patient charges you just entered. Change the Sort By field in the Claim Management window to Claim Number. Enter *10/29/2010* in both Transaction Dates boxes to create claims for that date only. Most offices transmit claims electronically; since this is not possible in this simulation, you will need to manually change the status of claims from Ready to Send to Sent after you create them.

8. Change the program date to November 1, 2010, since you will now begin entering some of today's transactions.

9. Set up patient accounts for two patients who had appointments with Dr. Yan this morning. Mr. and Mrs. Andrews will need to be entered as new patients. Use the Patient Information Forms shown in Source Documents 25 and 26 to record the patient information and to create cases for both patients. Refer to Source Documents 27 and 28 for each patient's diagnosis. Dr. Yan accepts assignment from Physician's Choice, which pays for 100 percent of covered services (Box A through Box H).

10. Enter the procedure charges and payments for the patients who had appointments this morning: Darla Andrews, Bill Andrews, Cedera Lomos, and Stanley Feldman (Source Documents 27–30). Print a walkout receipt for each patient who makes a payment. Be sure that the program date is set to Monday's date (11/1/2010) when you record the transactions.

- Use the existing case for Cedera Lomos since the reason for this visit is the same as the last visit.

- Create a new case for Stanley Feldman's visit.

11. Exit the Medisoft program, and make a backup copy of your data. Name the new file *PBsim1.mbk*.

Tuesday, November 2, 2010

Office closed for Election Day.

Wednesday, November 3, 2010

1. Remove Source Documents 31 through 42 on pages 245–267. Review the information provided on the source documents.

2. Start the Medisoft program, and restore the backup file from Monday, November 1, 2010 (PBsim1.mbk).

3. Set the program date to November 1, 2010, since you will start by entering the transactions from Monday afternoon. The office was closed on Tuesday, November 2, for Election Day.

4. Record the following transactions from Monday using the information provided on Source Documents 31–34. Use the Enter Transactions option to record the procedure charges and payments. Print a walkout receipt for each patient who makes a payment.

   - Enter the procedure charges and payment for Ethan Sampson (Source Document 31).

     Create a new case. Ethan is a full-time college student and is covered by his mother's (Caroline Sampson's) insurance (U.S. Life, Policy # 0123456, Group # R123, $15 copayment). Dr. Yan accepts assignment from U.S. Life, which pays 100 percent of covered services (Box A through Box H).

     Make sure the date for Ethan's procedures and copayment is 11/1/2010. Print a walkout receipt.

   - Enter the information and record the transactions for Jo Black, who is a new patient (Source Documents 32 and 33). Dr. Yan accepts assignment from Blue Cross and Blue Shield, which pays 80 percent of covered services (Box A through Box H). Jo has met her deductible.

   - Create a new case and record the transactions for Sarina Bell (Source Document 34). Be sure to enter and apply the copayment and print a walkout receipt.

5. A patient, James Smith, called the office to inquire about his account balance. Write the patient's account balance here: $_____

6. Process the remittance advice received from U.S. Life (Source Document 35). Use the Enter Deposits/Payments option.

   - When you apply the payment in the Apply Payment/Adjustments to Charges window, based on the RA:

     - Enter the Amt Paid Provider in the Payment field.

     - Enter the Allowed Amount in the Allowed field.

     - Tab to the end of the line.

     - When you are finished applying the payment for one patient, remember to save your work before selecting the next patient.

7. Print a patient day sheet for Monday, November 1, 2010. Enter *1/1/2000* and *1/1/2015* in the Date Created Range boxes, and enter *11/1/2010* in both Date From Range boxes. Be sure to check the box to show accounts receivable data at the end of the report.

8. Verify that you have entered the information correctly. The charges total $1,079.00, and the receipts total $−115.50. If these amounts do not match the information on the reports, find the error and make the necessary correction.

9. Create the insurance claims for the patient charges you just entered. Enter *11/1/2010* to create claims for that day only. Change the status of the claims from Ready to Send to Sent.

10. Change the program date to November 3, 2010, to enter today's transactions.

11. Process the transactions from this morning (Source Documents 36–42). Remember to print walkout receipts when required.

- Enter the procedure charge and payment for John Gardiner (Source Document 36).

  Create a new case. Gardiner is married and is employed full-time at the Stephenson Daily News. Gardiner's health insurance carrier is Physician's Choice (Policy # 6397008, Group # J10-32, $15 copayment). Dr. Yan accepts assignment from Physician's Choice, which pays 100 percent of covered services (Box A through Box H).

- Record the new telephone number for Paul Ramos (Source Document 37).

- Input the new patient information and create a new case for Sam Wu (Source Documents 38 and 39). Dr. Yan accepts assignment from U.S. Life, which pays 100 percent of covered services (Box A through Box H). Remember to complete the Condition tab in the Case window since this visit is for an automobile accident: In the top panel of the Condition tab, fill in the first two fields. In the Accident panel, fill in the Related To and State fields.

  Enter the procedures and copayment. Print a walkout receipt.

- Enter the transactions for Paul Ramos (Source Document 40).

  First, create a new case. Ramos is a full-time student, single, and currently not employed. He is covered by his mother's health insurance. Maritza Ramos and her son are insured with Physician's Choice (Policy # 33246A, Group # EF719, $15 copayment). Dr. Yan accepts assignment from Physician's Choice, which pays 100 percent of covered services (Box A through Box H).

- Record the procedure charge for Ellen Barmenstein (Source Document 41).

  Create a new case for this visit by copying one of her other cases.

- Record the procedure charge and copayment for Elizabeth Jones (Source Document 42). This visit is related to the previous acute sinusitis case.

12. Exit the Medisoft program, and make a backup copy of your data. Name the new file **PBsim2.mbk.**

Thursday, November 4, 2010

1. Remove and review Source Documents 43 through 53 on pages 269–289.

2. Start the Medisoft program, and restore the backup file from Wednesday, November 3, 2010 (PBsim2.mbk).

3. Set the program date to November 3, 2010, to enter the transactions from Wednesday afternoon.

4. Record the following transactions from Wednesday using the information provided on Source Documents 43–46. Print a walkout receipt for each patient who makes a payment.

   - Enter the procedure charges for James Smith (Source Document 43).

   - Record the transactions for Joe Abate, a new patient (Source Documents 44 and 45). Remember to enter 100 percent in the insurance coverage percent boxes.

   - Record the procedure charge for Sarabeth Smith (Source Document 46).

     Create a new case. Sarabeth, who is single, has her own insurance policy with Blue Cross and Blue Shield (Policy # 03467, Group # 2450, $250 deductible). Dr. Yan accepts assignment from Blue Cross and Blue Shield, which pays 80 percent of covered services (Box A through Box H). Sarabeth has met her deductible for 2010.

5. A patient, Jo Black, called the office to inquire about her account balance. Her insurance company has not paid on her claim yet, so you must tell her not to pay these amounts until her insurance has paid. Write the patient's total account balance here: $_____

   After Jo Black pays her $200 deductible, her insurance covers 80 percent of covered services, and she is responsible for the remaining 20 percent. Since she has met her deductible, what amount of the current balance is she responsible for? Write the amount here: $_____

6. Process the check from Marion Johnson that was received yesterday (Source Document 47) using the Transaction Entry window. Apply the payment to the oldest outstanding charges. *Note:* In the Apply Payment to Charges window, the amount the patient owes for each procedure is listed in the Balance column. To apply the payment, enter the amount displayed in the Balance column in the This Payment column for each procedure until the full amount is applied.

7. Enter the information on the remittance advice from U.S. Life (Source Document 48).

8. Enter the information on the remittance advice from Physician's Choice (Source Document 49).

9. Print a patient day sheet for Wednesday, November 3, 2010. Enter *1/1/2000* and *1/1/2015* in the Date Created Range boxes, and enter *11/3/2010* in both Date From Range boxes. Be sure to check the box to show accounts receivable data at the end of the report.

10. Verify that you have entered the information correctly so that you can prepare a bank deposit slip. The total charges are $1,257.00, and the total receipts are $−617.70. Make any necessary corrections.

11. Create insurance claims for the patient charges. Enter *11/3/2010* to create claims for that day only. Be sure to change the status of the newly created claims.

12. Change the program date to November 4, 2010, to enter today's transactions.

13. Process the transactions from this morning (Source Documents 50–52). Remember to print walkout receipts when required.

   • Enter the procedure charges for Maritza Ramos (Source Document 50).

      Create a new case. Maritza is a full-time employee of Sara's Dresses, and she is divorced. You will need to look at her son Paul's case to locate her insurance information.

      Enter the charges and copayment, and print a walkout receipt.

   • Create a new case, and then record the procedure charge and payment for Sarina Bell (Source Document 51).

   • Record the charge for Jo Wong (Source Document 52). This transaction is for her existing case.

14. Enter the information on the remittance advice from Blue Cross and Blue Shield (Source Document 53).

15. Exit the Medisoft program, and make a backup copy of your data. Name the new file *PBsim3.mbk.*

Friday, November 5, 2010

1. Remove and review Source Documents 54 through 59 on pages 291–301.

2. Start the Medisoft program, and restore the backup file from Thursday, November 4, 2010 (PBsim3.mbk).

3. Set the program date to November 4, 2010, to enter the transactions from Thursday afternoon.

4. Process the check from James L. Smith that was received yesterday (Source Document 54) using the Transaction Entry window. Apply the payment to the oldest outstanding charges.

5. Print a patient day sheet for Thursday, November 4, 2010. Enter *1/1/2000* and *1/1/2015* in the Date Created Range boxes, and enter *11/4/2010* in both Date From Range boxes. Be sure to check the box to show accounts receivable data at the end of the report.

6. Verify that you have entered the information correctly so that you can prepare a bank deposit slip. The charges total $119.00, and the receipts total $−412.40. Make any necessary corrections.

7. Create insurance claims for the patient charges. Enter *11/4/2010* to create claims for that day only. Change the status of the new claims to Sent.

8. Change the program date to November 5, 2010, to enter today's transactions.

9. Process the transactions from this morning (Source Documents 55–57). Remember to print walkout receipts when required.

   - Enter the procedure charges for Surendra Uzwahl, a new patient (Source Documents 55 and 56). Dr. Yan accepts assignment from Blue Cross and Blue Shield, which pays 80 percent of covered services (Box A through Box H). Surendra has met her deductible for 2010.

   - Record the transactions for Jonathan Bell (Source Document 57). He is a full-time student covered by his father's (Herbert Bell's) insurance.

10. Record and apply the payments from U.S. Life (Source Document 58) and Physician's Choice (Source Document 59).

11. Create remainder statements for patients with outstanding balances of $5.00 or more whose last names begin with *A* through *L*. Verify that the Sort By field in the Statement Management window is set to Statement Number. Four statements should be displayed to start with. When you create the new statements, enter *11/5/2010* in the second Transaction Dates box.

12. Print a remainder statement for Jo Black. For the report type, select Remainder Statements—All Payments. Enter Jo Black's chart number in both Chart Number Range boxes, and leave the remaining fields as they are. (Both Date From Range boxes should be blank.)

   - Change the status of all the remaining Batch 0 statements from Ready to Send to Sent using the Change Status button.

13. Print a Patient Aging Applied Payment report for all patients. Leave the default setting (1/1/1900) in the first Date From Range box, and enter *11/5/2010* in the second box.

14. Print a Practice Analysis report. Leave the default Date Created range, and use *10/29/2010* through *11/5/2010* for the Date From range. Be sure to check the box to show accounts receivable data at the end of the report.

15. Exit the Medisoft program, and make a backup copy of your data. Name the new file *PBsim4.mbk*.

16. Complete the Simulation Assessment Test if your instructor has provided you with a copy of it. Use the reports you printed during this session to answer the questions on the test.

Appendix: Office Hours

Introduction to Office Hours

Appointment scheduling is one of the most important tasks in a medical office. Different medical procedures take different lengths of time, and each appointment must be the right length. On the one hand, physicians want to be able to go from one appointment to another without unnecessary breaks. On the other hand, patients should not be kept waiting for a physician for more than a few minutes. Managing and juggling the schedule is usually the job of a medical office assistant working at the front desk. Medisoft provides a special program called Office Hours to handle appointment scheduling.

Overview of the Office Hours Window

The Office Hours program has its own window (see Figure A-1 on page 174), with its own menu bar and toolbar. The Office Hours menu bar lists the menus available: File, Edit, View, Lists, Reports, Tools, and Help. Under the menu bar is a toolbar with shortcut buttons. Office Hours functions are accessed by selecting an option from one of the menus or by clicking a button on the toolbar.

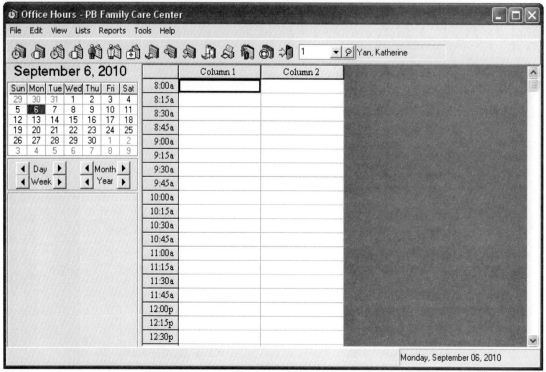

Figure A-1 *Office Hours Window*

Located just below the menu bar, the toolbar contains buttons that represent the most common activities performed in Office Hours. The name of each button is displayed when the cursor is placed over it. These buttons are shortcuts for frequently used menu commands. The toolbar displays fifteen buttons.

The left half of the Office Hours screen displays the current date and a calendar of the current month. The current date is highlighted on the calendar. When a different date is clicked on the calendar, the calendar switches the highlighting to the new date.

Note that Office Hours uses the computer's operating system date as the default date, not the Medisoft Program Date. For example, if you click the Go to Today button in Office Hours, the calendar will jump to the computer's operating system date rather than to the Medisoft Program Date. To change the date to the Medisoft Program Date, simply click that date on the calendar.

The Office Hours schedule, shown on the right half of the screen, is a listing of time slots for a particular day for a specific provider. The provider's name and number is displayed at the top to the right of the shortcut buttons. The provider can be easily changed by clicking the triangle button in the Provider box.

Program Options

When Office Hours is installed in a medical practice, it is set up to reflect the needs of that particular practice. Most offices that use Medisoft already have Office Hours set up and running. However, if Medisoft is just being installed, the options to set up the Office Hours program can be found in the Program Options dialog box, which is accessed by clicking Program Options on the Office Hours File menu.

Entering and Exiting Office Hours

Office Hours can be started from within Medisoft or directly from Windows. To access Office Hours from within Medisoft, click Appointment Book on the Activities menu. Office Hours can also be started by clicking the corresponding shortcut button on the Medisoft toolbar.

Follow these steps to start Office Hours without first entering Medisoft.

1. Click the Start button on the Windows task bar.

2. Click Medisoft on the Program submenu.

3. Click Office Hours on the Medisoft submenu.

The Office Hours program is closed by clicking Exit on the Office Hours File menu or by clicking the Exit button on the Office Hours toolbar. If Office Hours was started from within Medisoft, exiting will return you to Medisoft. If Office Hours was started directly from Windows, clicking Exit will return you to the Windows desktop.

Entering Appointments

Entering an appointment begins with selecting the provider for whom the appointment is being scheduled. The current provider is listed in the Provider box at the top right of the screen. Clicking the triangle button displays a drop-down list of providers in the system. To choose a different provider, click the name of the provider on the drop-down list.

After the provider is selected, the date of the desired appointment must be chosen. Dates are changed by clicking the Day, Week, Month, and Year right and left arrow buttons located under the calendar. After the provider and date have been selected, patient appointments can be entered.

Appointments are entered by clicking the Appointment Entry shortcut button or by double-clicking in a time slot on the schedule. When either of those actions is taken, the New Appointment Entry window is displayed (see Figure A-2). The window contains the following fields.

Chart A patient's chart number is chosen from the Chart drop-down list. To select the desired patient, click the name and press Enter. Once a patient's chart is selected from the Chart drop-down list, Medisoft displays the patient's name in the blank box to the right of the Chart box. If you are setting up an appointment for a new patient who has not been assigned a chart number, skip the Chart box and key the patient's name in the blank box to the right of the Chart box.

Phone After a patient's chart is selected, and the Tab or Enter key is pressed, that patient's phone number is automatically entered in the Phone box. If the appointment is for a new patient, the phone number can be entered manually.

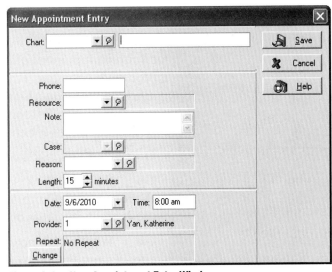

Figure A-2 *New Appointment Entry Window*

Resource This box is used if the practice assigns codes to resources, such as exam rooms or equipment.

Note Any special information about an appointment is entered in the Note box.

Case The case that pertains to the appointment is selected from the drop-down list of cases.

Reason Reason codes can be set up in the program to reflect the reason for an appointment, for example, a routine exam.

Length The amount of time an appointment will take (in minutes) is entered in the Length box by keying the number of minutes or by using the up and down arrows.

Date The Date box displays the date that is currently displayed on the calendar. If this is not the desired date, it may be changed by keying in a different date or by clicking the triangle button and using the pop-up calendar that appears.

Time The Time box displays the appointment time that is currently selected on the schedule. If this is not the desired time, it may be changed by keying a different time.

Provider The provider who will be treating the patient during this appointment is selected from the drop-down list of providers.

Repeat The Repeat box is used to enter appointments that recur on a regular basis.

After the boxes in the New Appointment Entry window have been completed, clicking the Save button enters the information on the schedule. The patient's name appears in the time slot corresponding to the appointment time. In addition, information about the appointment appears in the lower left corner of the Office Hours window.

Looking for a Future Date

Often a patient will need a follow-up appointment at a certain time in the future. For example, suppose a physician would like a patient to return for a checkup appointment in three weeks. The most efficient way to search for a future appointment in Office Hours is to use the Go to a Date shortcut button on the toolbar. This feature can also be accessed on the Edit menu.

Clicking the Go to a Date shortcut button (the eighth button from the left) displays the Go to Date window (see Figure A-3). Within the window, five boxes offer options for choosing a future date.

Date From This box indicates the current date in the appointment search.

Go __ Days This box is used to locate a date a specific number of days in the future. For example, if a patient needs an appointment ten days from the current day, *10* would be entered in this box.

Go __ Weeks This box is used when a patient needs an appointment a specific number of weeks in the future, such as six weeks from the current day.

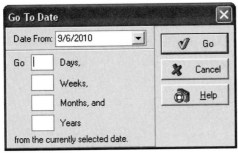

Figure A-3 *Go To Date Window*

Go __ Months This box is used when a patient needs an appointment a specific number of months in the future, such as three months from the current day.

Go __ Years This box is used when an appointment one year or several years in the future is needed.

After a number is entered in one or more of the boxes, clicking the Go button closes the window and begins the search. The system locates the future date and displays the calendar schedule for that date.

Computer Exercise A-1

Enter an appointment for Herbert Bell at 2:30 P.M. on Monday, September 6, 2010. The appointment is fifteen minutes in length and is with Dr. Katherine Yan.

1. Start Medisoft, and restore your latest backup file (for example, PBChap7.mbk or PBsim4.mbk). Click Appointment Book on the Medisoft Activities menu to open Office Hours.

2. Verify that *1—Yan, Katherine* is displayed in the Provider box.

3. Change the date on the calendar to Monday, September 6, 2010. Use the forward arrow keys to change the month and year, and then click the day in the calendar itself.

4. In the schedule, under Column 1, double-click the 2:30 P.M. time slot. (You may need to use the scroll bar to view 2:30 P.M.) The New Appointment Entry window is displayed.

5. Click *Herbert Bell* on the list of names on the drop-down list in the Chart box, and press Enter. The system automatically fills in a number of boxes in the window, such as the patient's name, phone number, and case.

6. Accept the default entry in the Case box.

7. Notice that the Length box already contains an entry of fifteen minutes. This is the default appointment length set up in Medisoft. Since Herbert Bell's appointment is for an annual exam, this entry must be changed to sixty minutes. Key *60* in the Length box, or use the up arrow next to the Length box to change the appointment length to sixty minutes.

$ BILLING TIP

The red X that appears next to the patient's name on the schedule is used in connection with the Eligibility Verification feature available on the Medisoft Activities menu. This feature, which is not used in this text, requires a special online connection and is used to verify a patient's insurance coverage.

8. Verify the entries in the Date, Time, and Provider boxes, and then click the Save button. Medisoft saves the appointment, closes the window, and displays the appointment on the schedule, as well as in the lower left corner of the Office Hours window. Herbert Bell's name is displayed in the 2:30 P.M. time slot on the schedule.

Computer Exercise A-2

Enter the following appointments for Dr. Katherine Yan.

1. The first appointment is Monday, September 6, 2010, at 3:30 P.M. for John Fitzwilliams, 30 minutes in length. Verify that *1—Yan, Katherine* is displayed in the Provider box.

2. On the schedule, double-click the 3:30 P.M. time slot.

3. Select *John Fitzwilliams* from the Chart drop-down list.

4. Press the Enter key. The program automatically completes several boxes in the window.

5. Press the Tab key until the entry in the Length box is highlighted.

6. Key *30* in the Length box, or click the up arrow once to change the length to thirty minutes.

7. Click the Save button. Verify that the appointment for John Fitzwilliams appears on the schedule for September 6, 2010, at 3:30 P.M. for a length of thirty minutes.

8. Enter an appointment on Monday, September 6, 2010, at 4:00 P.M. for Leila Patterson, 15 minutes in length.

9. Enter an appointment on Tuesday, September 7, 2010, at 1:30 P.M. for James Smith, 30 minutes in length.

10. Schedule an appointment two weeks after September 7, 2010, for James Smith at 12:15 P.M., 15 minutes in length. Click the Go To a Date shortcut button or select Go to Date on the Office Hours Edit menu.

11. Key *2* in the Go ___ Weeks box. Click the Go button. The program closes the Go To Date box and displays the cursor on the appointment schedule for September 21, 2010. Double-click in the 12:15 P.M. time slot.

12. Enter James Smith's appointment.

Computer Exercise A-3

Enter these appointments for Dr. Katherine Yan.

1. Verify that Dr. Katherine Yan is selected in the Provider drop-down box.

2. Enter an appointment for Tuesday, September 28, 2010, at 1:30 P.M. for Janine Bell, 15 minutes in length.

3. Use the Office Hours Go to a Date feature to schedule an appointment three weeks from September 28, 2010, at 2:30 P.M. for Sarina Bell, 30 minutes in length.

Searching for Available Appointment Time

Often it is necessary to search for available appointment space on a particular day of the week and at a specific time. For example, a patient needs a thirty-minute appointment during his lunch hour, which is from 12:00 P.M. to 1:00 P.M. He can get away from the office on Mondays and Fridays only. Office Hours makes it easy to locate an appointment slot that meets these requirements with the Search for Open Time Slot option.

Computer Exercise A-4

Search for the next available appointment slot beginning September 8, 2010, with Dr. Yan, on a Tuesday or Thursday, between 1:00 P.M. and 2:30 P.M.

1. Change the Office Hours calendar to September 8, 2010.

2. Verify that Dr. Katherine Yan is displayed in the Provider box.

3. On the Edit menu, click Find Open Time, or click the Search for Open Time Slot shortcut button. The Find Open Time window is displayed (see Figure A-4).

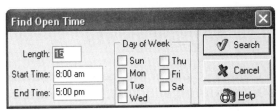

Figure A-4   *Find Open Time Window*

4. Enter *60* in the Length box. Press the Tab key.

5. Enter *1:00 pm* in the Start Time box.

6. Enter *2:30 pm* in the End Time box.

7. To search for an appointment on Tuesday or Thursday, click the Tuesday and Thursday boxes in the Day of Week area of the window.

8. Click the Search button to begin looking for an appointment slot. Medisoft closes the window and locates the first available time slot that meets these specifications. The time slot is outlined on the schedule.

9. Double-click the selected time slot. Click Maritza Ramos on the drop-down list in the Name box.

10. Press the Tab key until the cursor is in the Length box.

11. Key *60* and press the Tab key.

12. Click the Save button.

13. Verify that the appointment has been entered by looking at the schedule.

Entering Appointments for New Patients

When a new patient phones the office for an appointment, while the prospective patient is still on the phone, most offices obtain basic data and enter it in the appropriate Medisoft windows—the Patient/Guarantor window and the Case window. However, if necessary, the appointment can be scheduled in Office Hours before this information is entered in Medisoft.

Computer Exercise A-5

Schedule Lisa Green, a new patient, for a forty-five-minute appointment with Dr. Katherine Yan on September 28, 2010, at 1:45 P.M.

1. Go to September 28, 2010, on the schedule, and confirm that Dr. Yan is selected as the provider.

2. Double-click the 1:45 P.M. time slot

3. Click in the blank box to the right of the Chart box, and key *Green, Lisa.* Press the Tab key to move the cursor to the Phone box.

4. Key *6145553604* in the Phone box.

5. Key *45* in the Length box.

6. Click the Save button. Check to see that the appointment is displayed on the September 28, 2010, schedule.

Changing or Deleting Appointments

Very often it is necessary to change or cancel a patient's appointment. Changing an appointment is accomplished with the Cut and Paste commands on the Office Hours Edit menu.

The following steps are used to reschedule an appointment.

1. Locate the appointment that needs to be changed. Make sure the appointment slot is visible on the schedule.

2. Click the existing time slot. A black border surrounds the slot to indicate that it is selected.

3. Click Cut on the Edit menu. The appointment disappears from the schedule.

4. On the calendar, click the date on which the appointment is to be rescheduled.

5. Click the desired time slot on the schedule. The slot becomes active.

6. Click Paste on the Edit menu. The patient's name appears in the new time slot.

The following steps are used to cancel an appointment without rescheduling.

1. Locate the appointment on the schedule.

2. Click the time slot to select the appointment.

3. Click Cut on the Edit menu. The appointment disappears from the schedule.

Computer Exercise A-6

Reschedule Janine Bell's appointment.

1. Go to Tuesday, September 28, 2010, on the calendar.

2. Locate Janine Bell's 1:30 P.M. appointment on the schedule. Click the 1:30 P.M. time slot.

3. Click Cut on the Edit menu. (You may also use the right mouse click shortcut.) Janine Bell's appointment is removed from the 1:30 P.M. time slot.

4. Go to Thursday, September 30, 2010, and click the 3:00 P.M. time slot.

5. Click Paste on the Edit menu. Janine Bell's name is displayed in the 3:00 P.M. time slot for September 30, 2010.

Previewing and Printing Schedules

In most medical offices, providers' schedules are printed on a daily basis. To view a list of all appointments for a provider for a given day, click Appointment List on the Office Hours Reports menu. The report can be previewed on the screen or sent directly to the printer. If the preview option is selected, the appointment list is displayed in the standard Medisoft Preview Report window (see Figure A-5). The usual buttons on the toolbar can be used to view the schedule at different sizes, to move from page to page, and to print the schedule. Clicking the Close button closes the preview window.

The schedule can also be printed without using the Preview option by clicking the Print Appointment List shortcut button. Office Hours prints

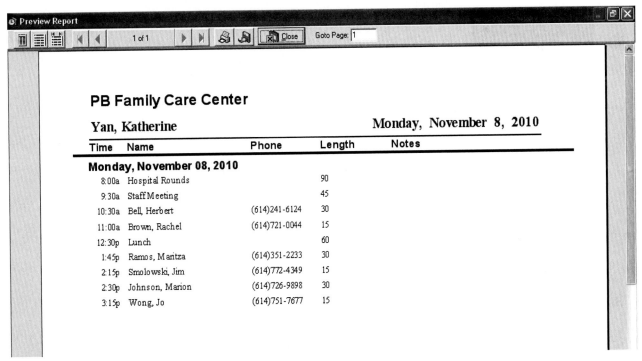

Figure A-5 *Preview Report Window*

the schedule for the provider who is listed in the Provider box. To print the schedule for a different provider, change the entry in the Provider box before printing the schedule.

Computer Exercise A-7

Print Dr. Katherine Yan's schedule for September 6, 2010.

1. Confirm that Dr. Katherine Yan is selected as the provider.

2. Go to Monday, September 6, 2010, on the calendar.

3. Click Appointment List on the Office Hours Reports menu. The Report Setup window appears.

4. Under Print Selection, click the button that sends the report directly to the printer, and then click the Start button.

5. The Data Selection window appears. Enter September 6, 2010, in both date boxes.

6. In both provider boxes, select 1 for Dr. Yan. Then click the OK button.

7. The Print window appears. Click OK to print the report.

8. Close the Office Hours program.

Computer Practice A-8: *Exiting the Program and Making a Backup Copy*

Exit the program, and create a backup copy of your work by following these steps.

1. Choose Exit from the File menu, or use the toolbar to select this option.

2. Click the Back Up Data Now button.

3. In the Destination File Path and Name box, enter the location where the backup file will be saved (if it is not already displayed). Name the new file *PBApp.mbk.*

4. Click the Start Backup button. When the Backup Complete box appears, click OK. The Medisoft program shuts down.

Source Documents

Use the Source Documents provided in this section to complete the tutorial (Source Documents 1–20, pages 185–223) and the simulation (Source Documents 21–59, pages 225–301).

PATIENT INFORMATION FORM

THIS SECTION REFERS TO PATIENT ONLY

Name: Juan Lomos	**Sex:** M **Marital Status:** ☐ S ☒ M ☐ D ☐ W **Birth Date:** 7/21/52
Address: 12 Briar Lane	**SS#:** 716-83-0061
City: Stephenson **State:** OH **Zip:** 60089	**Employer:** Stephenson Wire Works (full-time)
Home Phone: 614-221-0202	**Employer's Address:** 125 Stephenson Road
Work Phone: 614-525-0215	**City:** Stephenson **State:** OH **Zip:** 60089
Spouse's Name:	**Spouse's Employer:**
Emergency Contact:	**Relationship:** **Phone #:**

FILL IN IF PATIENT IS A MINOR

Parent/Guardian's Name:	**Sex:** **Marital Status:** ☐ S ☐ M ☐ D ☐ W **Birth Date:**
Phone:	**SS#:**
Address:	**Employer:**
City: **State:** **Zip:**	**Employer's Address:**
Student Status:	**City:** **State:** **Zip:**

INSURANCE INFORMATION

Primary Insurance Company: Blue Cross Blue Shield	**Secondary Insurance Company:**
Subscriber's Name: Juan Lomos **Birth Date:** 7/21/52	**Subscriber's Name:** **Birth Date:**
Plan: Traditional **SS#:** 716-83-0061	**Plan:**
Policy #: 716830061 **Group #:** 126	**Policy #:** **Group #:**
Copayment: **Deductible:** $250 **Price Code:** A	

OTHER INFORMATION

Reason for visit: Auto accident--back injury	**Allergy to Medication (list):**
Name of referring physician:	**If auto accident, list date and state in which it occurred:** OH -- 8/8/10

I authorize treatment and agree to pay all fees and charges for the person named above. I agree to pay all charges shown by statements, promptly upon their presentation, unless credit arrangements are agreed upon in writing.

I authorize payment directly to **FAMILY CARE CENTER** of insurance benefits otherwise payable to me. I hereby authorize the release of any medical information necessary in order to process a claim for payment in my behalf.

Juan Lomos	9/3/10
(Patient's Signature/Parent or Guardian's Signature)	(Date)

I plan to make payment of my medical expenses as follows (check one or more):

___X___ Insurance (as above)   ___X___ Cash/Check/Credit/Debit Card   _____ Medicare   _____ Medicaid   _____ Workers' Comp.

Family Care Center
285 Stephenson Boulevard
Stephenson, OH 60089
614-555-0100

From the Desk of Dr. Katherine Yan

Date   9/3/2010

Patient   Juan Lomos

Physician's Notes

Condition related to automobile accident in Ohio on 8/8/10

Patient was hospitalized from 8/8/10 to 8/14/10

Patient was totally disabled from 8/8/10 to 8/19/10

Patient was partially disabled from 8/20/10 to 9/1/10.

PATIENT INFORMATION FORM

THIS SECTION REFERS TO PATIENT ONLY

Name: Cedera Lomos	Sex: F	Marital Status: ☐S ☒M ☐D ☐W	Birth Date: 5/21/57

Address: 12 Briar Lane	SS#: 717-87-0054

City: Stephenson	State: OH	Zip: 60089	Employer: The Oyster Bar (full-time)

Home Phone: 614-221-0202	Employer's Address:

Work Phone: 614-299-0313	City: Stephenson	State: OH	Zip: 60089

Spouse's Name:	Spouse's Employer:

Emergency Contact:	Relationship:	Phone #:

FILL IN IF PATIENT IS A MINOR

Parent/Guardian's Name:	Sex:	Marital Status: ☐S ☐M ☐D ☐W	Birth Date:

Phone:	SS#:

Address:	Employer:

City:	State:	Zip:	Employer's Address:

Student Status:	City:	State:	Zip:

INSURANCE INFORMATION

Primary Insurance Company: Blue Cross/Blue Shield	Secondary Insurance Company: Physician's Alliance of Ohio

Subscriber's Name: Juan Lomos	Birth Date: 7/21/52	Rel. to Insured spouse	Subscriber's Name: Cedera Lomos	Birth Date: 5/21/57	Rel. to Insured self

Plan: Traditional	SS#: 716-83-0061	Plan: Traditional	SS#: 717-87-0054

Policy #: 716830061	Group #: 126	Policy #: 621382	Group #: A435

Copayment:	Deductible: $250	Price Code: A	Copayment:	Deductible: $100	Price Code: A

OTHER INFORMATION

Reason for visit: Persistent cough	Allergy to Medication (list): penicillin

Name of referring physician:	If auto accident, list date and state in which it occurred:

I authorize treatment and agree to pay all fees and charges for the person named above. I agree to pay all charges shown by statements, promptly upon their presentation, unless credit arrangements are agreed upon in writing.

I authorize payment directly to FAMILY CARE CENTER of insurance benefits otherwise payable to me. I hereby authorize the release of any medical information necessary in order to process a claim for payment in my behalf.

Cedera Lomos	9/3/10
(Patient's Signature/Parent or Guardian's Signature)	(Date)

I plan to make payment of my medical expenses as follows (check one or more):

_X_ Insurance (as above)   _X_ Cash/Check/Credit/Debit Card   ____ Medicare   ____ Medicaid   ____ Workers' Comp.

PATIENT INFORMATION FORM

THIS SECTION REFERS TO PATIENT ONLY

Name: Lisa Lomos	Sex: F	Marital Status: ☒S ☐M ☐D ☐W	Birth Date: 6/3/04

Address: 12 Briar Lane	SS#: 212-55-3311

City: Stephenson	State: OH	Zip: 60089	Employer:

Home Phone: 614-221-0202	Employer's Address:

Work Phone:	City:	State:	Zip:

Spouse's Name:	Spouse's Employer:

Emergency Contact:	Relationship:	Phone #:

FILL IN IF PATIENT IS A MINOR

Parent/Guardian's Name: Juan Lomos	Sex: M	Marital Status: ☐S ☒M ☐D ☐W	Birth Date: 7/21/52

Phone: 614-221-0202	SS#: 716-83-0061

Address: 12 Briar Lane	Employer: Stephenson Wire Works

City: Stephenson	State: OH	Zip: 60089	Employer's Address: 125 Stephenson Road

Student Status: full-time	City: Stephenson	State: OH	Zip: 60089

INSURANCE INFORMATION

Primary Insurance Company: Blue Cross/Blue Shield	Secondary Insurance Company: Physician's Alliance of Ohio

Subscriber's Name: Juan Lomos	Birth Date: 7/21/52	Rel. to Insured child	Subscriber's Name: Cedera Lomos	Birth Date: 5/21/57	Rel. to Insured child

Plan: Traditional	SS#: 716-83-0061	Plan: Traditional	SS#: 717-87-0054

Policy #: 716830061	Group #: 126	Policy #: 621382	Group #: A435

Copayment:	Deductible: $250	Price Code: A	Copayment:	Deductible: $100	Price Code: A

OTHER INFORMATION

Reason for visit: Routine well-child checkup	Allergy to Medication (list):

Name of referring physician:	If auto accident, list date and state in which it occurred:

I authorize treatment and agree to pay all fees and charges for the person named above. I agree to pay all charges shown by statements, promptly upon their presentation, unless credit arrangements are agreed upon in writing.

I authorize payment directly to FAMILY CARE CENTER of insurance benefits otherwise payable to me. I hereby authorize the release of any medical information necessary in order to process a claim for payment in my behalf.

Juan Lomos   9/3/10

(Patient's Signature/Parent or Guardian's Signature)   (Date)

I plan to make payment of my medical expenses as follows (check one or more):

__X__ Insurance (as above)   __X__ Cash/Check/Credit/Debit Card   ____ Medicare   ____ Medicaid   ____ Workers' Comp.

PATIENT INFORMATION FORM

THIS SECTION REFERS TO PATIENT ONLY

Name: Angela Wong	Sex: F	Marital Status: ☒S ☐M ☐D ☐W	Birth Date: 3/8/92

Address: 10 Maytime Lane, Apt. 3	SS#: 123-62-2111

City: Stephenson	State: OH	Zip: 60089	Employer:

Home Phone: 614-212-0808	Employer's Address:

Work Phone:	City:	State:	Zip:

Spouse's Name:	Spouse's Employer:

Emergency Contact:	Relationship:	Phone #:

FILL IN IF PATIENT IS A MINOR

Parent/Guardian's Name: Peter Wong	Sex: M	Marital Status: ☐S ☐M ☒D ☐W	Birth Date: 1/17/62

Phone: 614-212-0496	SS#: 419-83-7756

Address: 320 Fourth Street	Employer: U.S. Army (full-time)

City: Stephenson	State: OH	Zip: 60089	Employer's Address: 100 North Andover Road

Student Status: full-time	City: Stephenson	State: OH	Zip: 60089

INSURANCE INFORMATION

Primary Insurance Company: Tricare	Secondary Insurance Company:

Subscriber's Name: Peter Wong	Birth Date: 1/17/62	Rel. to Insured child	Subscriber's Name:	Birth Date:	Rel. to Insured

Plan: Tricare	SS#: 419-83-7756	Plan:	SS#:

Policy #: 397214A	Group #: 647	Policy #:	Group #:

Copayment: $10	Deductible:	Price Code: A	Copayment:	Deductible:	Price Code:

OTHER INFORMATION

Reason for visit: Checkup	Allergy to Medication (list):

Name of referring physician:	If auto accident, list date and state in which it occurred:

I authorize treatment and agree to pay all fees and charges for the person named above. I agree to pay all charges shown by statements, promptly upon their presentation, unless credit arrangements are agreed upon in writing.

I authorize payment directly to FAMILY CARE CENTER of insurance benefits otherwise payable to me. I hereby authorize the release of any medical information necessary in order to process a claim for payment in my behalf.

Peter Wong	9/3/10
(Patient's Signature/Parent or Guardian's Signature)	(Date)

I plan to make payment of my medical expenses as follows (check one or more):

__X__ Insurance (as above)   __X__ Cash/Check/Credit/Debit Card   _____ Medicare   _____ Medicaid   _____ Workers' Comp.

Family Care Center
285 Stephenson Boulevard
Stephenson, OH 60089
614-555-0100

Date 9/3/2010

John Fitzwilliams' New Employer

Jenny Designs (full-time)

Family Care Center
285 Stephenson Boulevard
Stephenson, OH 60089
614-555-0100

From the Desk of Dr. Katherine Yan

Date   **9/3/2010**

Patient   **Herbert Mitchell**

Physician's Notes

Patient was hospitalized for angina from 8/8/2010 through 8/10/2010.

Medicare representative was contacted and authorized treatment.
Authorization number is 128-33821.

ENCOUNTER FORM

9/3/10   **10:30am**
DATE   TIME

Dr. Katherine Yan
PROVIDER

Cedera Lomos
PATIENT NAME

LOMCE000
CHART #

OFFICE VISITS - SYMPTOMATIC - NEW		
99201	OF--New Patient Minimal	
99202	OF--New Patient Low	
99203	OF--New Patient Detailed	
99204	OF--New Patient Moderate	X
99205	OF--New Patient High	
OFFICE VISITS - SYMPTOMATIC - ESTABLISHED		
99211	OF--Established Patient Minimal	
99212	OF--Established Patient Low	
99213	OF--Established Patient Detailed	
99214	OF--Established Patient Moderate	
99215	OF--Established Patient High	
PREVENTIVE VISITS - NEW		
99381	Under 1 Year	
99382	1 - 4 Years	
99383	5 - 11 Years	
99384	12 - 17 Years	
99385	18 - 39 Years	
99386	40 - 64 Years	
99387	65 Years & Up	
PREVENTIVE VISITS - ESTABLISHED		
99391	Under 1 Year	
99392	1 - 4 Years	
99393	5 - 11 Years	
99394	12 - 17 Years	
99395	18 - 39 Years	
99396	40 - 64 Years	
99397	65 Years & Up	
PROCEDURES		
12011	Repair of superficial wounds, face	
29125	Short arm splint	
45378	Colonoscopy--diagnostic	
45380	Colonoscopy--biopsy	
71010	Chest x-ray, frontal	
71020	Chest x-ray, frontal and lateral	
73070	Elbow x-ray, AP and lateral	

PROCEDURES		
73090	Forearm x-ray, AP and lateral	
73100	Wrist x-ray, AP and lateral	
73600	Ankle x-ray, AP and lateral	
93000	Electrocardiogram--ECG	
93015	Treadmill stress test	
LABORATORY		
80061	Lipid panel	
82270	Hemoccult--stool screening	
82465	Cholesterol test	
82947	Glucose--quantitative	
82951	Glucose tolerance test	
83718	HDL cholesterol test	
85007	Manual WBC	
85025	CBC w/diff.	
85651	Erythrocyte sed rate--ESR	
86580	Mantoux test	
87040	Bacterial culture	
87430	Strep screen	
87086	Urine colony count	
87088	Urine culture	
INJECTIONS		
90465	Immunization administration, pt under 8 yrs	
90471	Immunization administration	
90657	Influenza injection, under 35 months	
90658	Influenza injection, older than 3 years	
90703	Tetanus immunization	
90707	MMR immunization	

PB FAMILY CARE CENTER		NOTES
REFERRING PHYSICIAN	NPI	
AUTHORIZATION #		
DIAGNOSIS **473.9 Chronic sinusitis**		
PAYMENT AMOUNT		

ENCOUNTER FORM

9/3/10 11:00am	Dr. Katherine Yan
DATE TIME	PROVIDER
Lisa Lomos	LOMLI000
PATIENT NAME	CHART #

OFFICE VISITS - SYMPTOMATIC - NEW		
99201	OF--New Patient Minimal	
99202	OF--New Patient Low	
99203	OF--New Patient Detailed	
99204	OF--New Patient Moderate	
99205	OF--New Patient High	

OFFICE VISITS - SYMPTOMATIC - ESTABLISHED		
99211	OF--Established Patient Minimal	
99212	OF--Established Patient Low	
99213	OF--Established Patient Detailed	
99214	OF--Established Patient Moderate	
99215	OF--Established Patient High	

PREVENTIVE VISITS - NEW		
99381	Under 1 Year	
99382	1 - 4 Years	
99383	5 - 11 Years	X
99384	12 - 17 Years	
99385	18 - 39 Years	
99386	40 - 64 Years	
99387	65 Years & Up	

PREVENTIVE VISITS - ESTABLISHED		
99391	Under 1 Year	
99392	1 - 4 Years	
99393	5 - 11 Years	
99394	12 - 17 Years	
99395	18 - 39 Years	
99396	40 - 64 Years	
99397	65 Years & Up	

PROCEDURES		
12011	Repair of superficial wounds, face	
29125	Short arm splint	
45378	Colonoscopy--diagnostic	
45380	Colonoscopy--biopsy	
71010	Chest x-ray, frontal	
71020	Chest x-ray, frontal and lateral	
73070	Elbow x-ray, AP and lateral	

PROCEDURES		
73090	Forearm x-ray, AP and lateral	
73100	Wrist x-ray, AP and lateral	
73600	Ankle x-ray, AP and lateral	
93000	Electrocardiogram--ECG	
93015	Treadmill stress test	

LABORATORY		
80061	Lipid panel	
82270	Hemoccult--stool screening	
82465	Cholesterol test	
82947	Glucose--quantitative	
82951	Glucose tolerance test	
83718	HDL cholesterol test	
85007	Manual WBC	
85025	CBC w/diff.	
85651	Erythrocyte sed rate--ESR	
86580	Mantoux test	
87040	Bacterial culture	
87430	Strep screen	
87086	Urine colony count	
87088	Urine culture	

INJECTIONS		
90465	Immunization administration, pt under 8 yrs	
90471	Immunization administration	
90657	Influenza injection, under 35 months	
90658	Influenza injection, older than 3 years	
90703	Tetanus immunization	
90707	MMR immunization	

PB FAMILY CARE CENTER		NOTES
REFERRING PHYSICIAN	NPI	
AUTHORIZATION #		
DIAGNOSIS		
v20.2 health checkup		
PAYMENT AMOUNT		

ENCOUNTER FORM

9/3/10	11:30am	Dr. Katherine Yan
DATE	TIME	PROVIDER

Leila Patterson	PATLE000
PATIENT NAME	CHART #

OFFICE VISITS - SYMPTOMATIC - NEW		
99201	OF--New Patient Minimal	
99202	OF--New Patient Low	
99203	OF--New Patient Detailed	
99204	OF--New Patient Moderate	
99205	OF--New Patient High	
OFFICE VISITS - SYMPTOMATIC - ESTABLISHED		
99211	OF--Established Patient Minimal	
99212	OF--Established Patient Low	X
99213	OF--Established Patient Detailed	
99214	OF--Established Patient Moderate	
99215	OF--Established Patient High	
PREVENTIVE VISITS - NEW		
99381	Under 1 Year	
99382	1 - 4 Years	
99383	5 - 11 Years	
99384	12 - 17 Years	
99385	18 - 39 Years	
99386	40 - 64 Years	
99387	65 Years & Up	
PREVENTIVE VISITS - ESTABLISHED		
99391	Under 1 Year	
99392	1 - 4 Years	
99393	5 - 11 Years	
99394	12 - 17 Years	
99395	18 - 39 Years	
99396	40 - 64 Years	
99397	65 Years & Up	
PROCEDURES		
12011	Repair of superficial wounds, face	
29125	Short arm splint	
45378	Colonoscopy--diagnostic	
45380	Colonoscopy--biopsy	
71010	Chest x-ray, frontal	
71020	Chest x-ray, frontal and lateral	
73070	Elbow x-ray, AP and lateral	

PROCEDURES		
73090	Forearm x-ray, AP and lateral	
73100	Wrist x-ray, AP and lateral	
73600	Ankle x-ray, AP and lateral	
93000	Electrocardiogram--ECG	
93015	Treadmill stress test	
LABORATORY		
80061	Lipid panel	
82270	Hemoccult--stool screening	
82465	Cholesterol test	X
82947	Glucose--quantitative	
82951	Glucose tolerance test	
83718	HDL cholesterol test	
85007	Manual WBC	
85025	CBC w/diff.	
85651	Erythrocyte sed rate--ESR	
86580	Mantoux test	
87040	Bacterial culture	
87430	Strep screen	
87086	Urine colony count	
87088	Urine culture	
INJECTIONS		
90465	Immunization administration, pt under 8 yrs	
90471	Immunization administration	
90657	Influenza injection, under 35 months	
90658	Influenza injection, older than 3 years	
90703	Tetanus immunization	
90707	MMR immunization	

PB FAMILY CARE CENTER		NOTES
REFERRING PHYSICIAN	NPI	
AUTHORIZATION #		
DIAGNOSIS 272.0 hypercholesterolemia		
PAYMENT AMOUNT		

PATIENT INFORMATION FORM

THIS SECTION REFERS TO PATIENT ONLY

Name: Leila Patterson		Sex: F	Marital Status: ☒S ☐M ☐D ☐W	Birth Date: 2/14/49

Address: 2 Woods Street

SS#: 813-22-9549

City: Jefferson	State: OH	Zip: 60093	Employer:

Home Phone: 614-626-2099

Employer's Address:

Work Phone:	City:	State:	Zip:

Spouse's Name:

Spouse's Employer:

Emergency Contact:	Relationship:	Phone #:

FILL IN IF PATIENT IS A MINOR

Parent/Guardian's Name:	Sex:	Marital Status: ☐S ☐M ☐D ☐W	Birth Date:

Phone:

SS#:

Address:

Employer:

City:	State:	Zip:	Employer's Address:

Student Status:	City:	State:	Zip:

INSURANCE INFORMATION

Primary Insurance Company: Oxford	Secondary Insurance Company:

Subscriber's Name: self	Birth Date:	Rel. to Insured	Subscriber's Name:	Birth Date:	Rel. to Insured

Plan: Liberty	SS#:	Plan:	SS#:

Policy #: L813229549	Group #:	Policy #:	Group #:

Copayment:	Deductible: $500 (met)	Price Code: A	Copayment:	Deductible:	Price Code:

OTHER INFORMATION

Reason for visit: Cholesterol check	Allergy to Medication (list):

Name of referring physician:	If auto accident, list date and state in which it occurred:

I authorize treatment and agree to pay all fees and charges for the person named above. I agree to pay all charges shown by statements, promptly upon their presentation, unless credit arrangements are agreed upon in writing.

I authorize payment directly to FAMILY CARE CENTER of insurance benefits otherwise payable to me. I hereby authorize the release of any medical information necessary in order to process a claim for payment in my behalf.

Leila Patterson	9/3/10
(Patient's Signature/Parent or Guardian's Signature)	(Date)

I plan to make payment of my medical expenses as follows (check one or more):

__X__ Insurance (as above) __X__ Cash/Check/Credit/Debit Card _____ Medicare _____ Medicaid _____ Workers' Comp.

Family Care Center
285 Stephenson Boulevard
Stephenson, OH 60089
614-555-0100

New Insurance Carrier: Oxford

Address Tab

Code: 13

Name: Oxford

Street: 100 Colony Ct.

City: Cincinnati

State: OH

Zip: 60314

Phone: 614-555-0014

Practice ID: 02385496

Options Tab

Plan Name: Liberty

Type: Other

☒ Delay Secondary Billing

Patient Signature on File: Signature on File

Insured Signature on File: Signature on File

Physician Signature on File: Signature on File

Print PINs on Forms: Leave Blank

Default Billing Method: Electronic

EDI/Eligibility Tab

EDI Receiver: Phoenix

NDC Record Code: 01

ENCOUNTER FORM

9/3/10   12:00pm
DATE   TIME

Dr. Katherine Yan
PROVIDER

Ellen Barmenstein
PATIENT NAME

BAREL000
CHART #

OFFICE VISITS - SYMPTOMATIC - NEW		
99201	OF--New Patient Minimal	
99202	OF--New Patient Low	
99203	OF--New Patient Detailed	
99204	OF--New Patient Moderate	
99205	OF--New Patient High	
OFFICE VISITS - SYMPTOMATIC - ESTABLISHED		
99211	OF--Established Patient Minimal	X
99212	OF--Established Patient Low	
99213	OF--Established Patient Detailed	
99214	OF--Established Patient Moderate	
99215	OF--Established Patient High	
PREVENTIVE VISITS - NEW		
99381	Under 1 Year	
99382	1 - 4 Years	
99383	5 - 11 Years	
99384	12 - 17 Years	
99385	18 - 39 Years	
99386	40 - 64 Years	
99387	65 Years & Up	
PREVENTIVE VISITS - ESTABLISHED		
99391	Under 1 Year	
99392	1 - 4 Years	
99393	5 - 11 Years	
99394	12 - 17 Years	
99395	18 - 39 Years	
99396	40 - 64 Years	
99397	65 Years & Up	
PROCEDURES		
12011	Repair of superficial wounds, face	
29125	Short arm splint	
45378	Colonoscopy--diagnostic	
45380	Colonoscopy--biopsy	
71010	Chest x-ray, frontal	
71020	Chest x-ray, frontal and lateral	
73070	Elbow x-ray, AP and lateral	

PROCEDURES		
73090	Forearm x-ray, AP and lateral	
73100	Wrist x-ray, AP and lateral	
73600	Ankle x-ray, AP and lateral	
93000	Electrocardiogram--ECG	
93015	Treadmill stress test	
LABORATORY		
80061	Lipid panel	
82270	Hemoccult--stool screening	
82465	Cholesterol test	
82947	Glucose--quantitative	
82951	Glucose tolerance test	
83718	HDL cholesterol test	
85007	Manual WBC	
85025	CBC w/diff.	
85651	Erythrocyte sed rate--ESR	
86580	Mantoux test	
87040	Bacterial culture	
87430	Strep screen	
87086	Urine colony count	
87088	Urine culture	
INJECTIONS		
90465	Immunization administration, pt under 8 yrs	
90471	Immunization administration	X
90657	Influenza injection, under 35 months	
90658	Influenza injection, older than 3 years	X
90703	Tetanus immunization	
90707	MMR immunization	

PB FAMILY CARE CENTER		NOTES
REFERRING PHYSICIAN	NPI	
AUTHORIZATION #		
DIAGNOSIS		
v04.81 Immunization -- flu		
PAYMENT AMOUNT		

ENCOUNTER FORM

9/3/10	**12:30pm**
DATE	TIME

Hiro Tanaka
PATIENT NAME

Dr. Katherine Yan
PROVIDER

TANHI000
CHART #

OFFICE VISITS - SYMPTOMATIC - NEW		
99201	OF--New Patient Minimal	
99202	OF--New Patient Low	
99203	OF--New Patient Detailed	
99204	OF--New Patient Moderate	
99205	OF--New Patient High	
OFFICE VISITS - SYMPTOMATIC - ESTABLISHED		
99211	OF--Established Patient Minimal	
99212	OF--Established Patient Low	X
99213	OF--Established Patient Detailed	
99214	OF--Established Patient Moderate	
99215	OF--Established Patient High	
PREVENTIVE VISITS - NEW		
99381	Under 1 Year	
99382	1 - 4 Years	
99383	5 - 11 Years	
99384	12 - 17 Years	
99385	18 - 39 Years	
99386	40 - 64 Years	
99387	65 Years & Up	
PREVENTIVE VISITS - ESTABLISHED		
99391	Under 1 Year	
99392	1 - 4 Years	
99393	5 - 11 Years	
99394	12 - 17 Years	
99395	18 - 39 Years	
99396	40 - 64 Years	
99397	65 Years & Up	
PROCEDURES		
12011	Repair of superficial wounds, face	
29125	Short arm splint	
45378	Colonoscopy--diagnostic	
45380	Colonoscopy--biopsy	
71010	Chest x-ray, frontal	
71020	Chest x-ray, frontal and lateral	
73070	Elbow x-ray, AP and lateral	

PROCEDURES		
73090	Forearm x-ray, AP and lateral	
73100	Wrist x-ray, AP and lateral	
73600	Ankle x-ray, AP and lateral	
93000	Electrocardiogram--ECG	
93015	Treadmill stress test	
LABORATORY		
80061	Lipid panel	
82270	Hemoccult--stool screening	
82465	Cholesterol test	
82947	Glucose--quantitative	
82951	Glucose tolerance test	
83718	HDL cholesterol test	
85007	Manual WBC	
85025	CBC w/diff.	
85651	Erythrocyte sed rate--ESR	
86580	Mantoux test	
87040	Bacterial culture	
87430	Strep screen	
87086	Urine colony count	
87088	Urine culture	
INJECTIONS		
90465	Immunization administration, pt under 8 yrs	
90471	Immunization administration	
90657	Influenza injection, under 35 months	
90658	Influenza injection, older than 3 years	
90703	Tetanus immunization	
90707	MMR immunization	

PB FAMILY CARE CENTER		NOTES
REFERRING PHYSICIAN	NPI	
AUTHORIZATION #		
DIAGNOSIS		
848.9 sprain or strain		
PAYMENT AMOUNT		
$10 copayment, check #3022		

ENCOUNTER FORM

9/3/10	1:00pm	Dr. Katherine Yan
DATE	TIME	PROVIDER

Elizabeth Jones	JONEL000
PATIENT NAME	CHART #

OFFICE VISITS - SYMPTOMATIC - NEW		
99201	OF--New Patient Minimal	
99202	OF--New Patient Low	
99203	OF--New Patient Detailed	
99204	OF--New Patient Moderate	
99205	OF--New Patient High	
OFFICE VISITS - SYMPTOMATIC - ESTABLISHED		
99211	OF--Established Patient Minimal	
99212	OF--Established Patient Low	X
99213	OF--Established Patient Detailed	
99214	OF--Established Patient Moderate	
99215	OF--Established Patient High	
PREVENTIVE VISITS - NEW		
99381	Under 1 Year	
99382	1 - 4 Years	
99383	5 - 11 Years	
99384	12 - 17 Years	
99385	18 - 39 Years	
99386	40 - 64 Years	
99387	65 Years & Up	
PREVENTIVE VISITS - ESTABLISHED		
99391	Under 1 Year	
99392	1 - 4 Years	
99393	5 - 11 Years	
99394	12 - 17 Years	
99395	18 - 39 Years	
99396	40 - 64 Years	
99397	65 Years & Up	
PROCEDURES		
12011	Repair of superficial wounds, face	
29125	Short arm splint	
45378	Colonoscopy--diagnostic	
45380	Colonoscopy--biopsy	
71010	Chest x-ray, frontal	
71020	Chest x-ray, frontal and lateral	
73070	Elbow x-ray, AP and lateral	

PROCEDURES		
73090	Forearm x-ray, AP and lateral	
73100	Wrist x-ray, AP and lateral	
73600	Ankle x-ray, AP and lateral	
93000	Electrocardiogram--ECG	
93015	Treadmill stress test	
LABORATORY		
80061	Lipid panel	
82270	Hemoccult--stool screening	
82465	Cholesterol test	
82947	Glucose--quantitative	
82951	Glucose tolerance test	
83718	HDL cholesterol test	
85007	Manual WBC	
85025	CBC w/diff.	
85651	Erythrocyte sed rate--ESR	
86580	Mantoux test	
87040	Bacterial culture	
87430	Strep screen	
87086	Urine colony count	
87088	Urine culture	
INJECTIONS		
90465	Immunization administration, pt under 8 yrs	
90471	Immunization administration	
90657	Influenza injection, under 35 months	
90658	Influenza injection, older than 3 years	
90703	Tetanus immunization	
90707	MMR immunization	

PB FAMILY CARE CENTER		NOTES
REFERRING PHYSICIAN	NPI	
AUTHORIZATION #		
DIAGNOSIS		
461.9 Acute sinusitis		
PAYMENT AMOUNT		
$15 copayment, check #609		

ENCOUNTER FORM

9/3/10	1:30pm	Dr. Katherine Yan
DATE	TIME	PROVIDER

Sarina Bell	BELSA001
PATIENT NAME	CHART #

OFFICE VISITS - SYMPTOMATIC - NEW		
99201	OF--New Patient Minimal	
99202	OF--New Patient Low	
99203	OF--New Patient Detailed	
99204	OF--New Patient Moderate	
99205	OF--New Patient High	
OFFICE VISITS - SYMPTOMATIC - ESTABLISHED		
99211	OF--Established Patient Minimal	
99212	OF--Established Patient Low	X
99213	OF--Established Patient Detailed	
99214	OF--Established Patient Moderate	
99215	OF--Established Patient High	
PREVENTIVE VISITS - NEW		
99381	Under 1 Year	
99382	1 - 4 Years	
99383	5 - 11 Years	
99384	12 - 17 Years	
99385	18 - 39 Years	
99386	40 - 64 Years	
99387	65 Years & Up	
PREVENTIVE VISITS - ESTABLISHED		
99391	Under 1 Year	
99392	1 - 4 Years	
99393	5 - 11 Years	
99394	12 - 17 Years	
99395	18 - 39 Years	
99396	40 - 64 Years	
99397	65 Years & Up	
PROCEDURES		
12011	Repair of superficial wounds, face	
29125	Short arm splint	
45378	Colonoscopy--diagnostic	
45380	Colonoscopy--biopsy	
71010	Chest x-ray, frontal	
71020	Chest x-ray, frontal and lateral	
73070	Elbow x-ray, AP and lateral	

PROCEDURES		
73090	Forearm x-ray, AP and lateral	
73100	Wrist x-ray, AP and lateral	
73600	Ankle x-ray, AP and lateral	
93000	Electrocardiogram--ECG	
93015	Treadmill stress test	
LABORATORY		
80061	Lipid panel	
82270	Hemoccult--stool screening	
82465	Cholesterol test	
82947	Glucose--quantitative	
82951	Glucose tolerance test	
83718	HDL cholesterol test	
85007	Manual WBC	
85025	CBC w/diff.	X
85651	Erythrocyte sed rate--ESR	
86580	Mantoux test	
87040	Bacterial culture	
87430	Strep screen	X
87086	Urine colony count	
87088	Urine culture	
INJECTIONS		
90465	Immunization administration, pt under 8 yrs	
90471	Immunization administration	
90657	Influenza injection, under 35 months	
90658	Influenza injection, older than 3 years	
90703	Tetanus immunization	
90707	MMR immunization	

PB FAMILY CARE CENTER		NOTES
REFERRING PHYSICIAN	NPI	
AUTHORIZATION #		
DIAGNOSIS 034.0 strep sore throat		
PAYMENT AMOUNT $15 copayment, check #309		

BLUE CROSS BLUE SHIELD
340 Preston Boulevard
Columbus, OH 60220

PROVIDER REMITTANCE
THIS IS NOT A BILL
A PAYMENT SUMMARY AND AN EXPLANATION OF
CODES ARE AT THE END OF THIS STATEMENT

FAMILY CARE CENTER
285 STEPHENSON BLVD.
STEPHENSON, OH 60089

Date Prepared:	9/7/10
EFT Number:	36094251
Amount:	$ 575.20

PROVIDER: KATHERINE YAN, M.D.

PATIENT: FELDMAN, STANLEY

PROC CODE	Date of Service From–Thru	Qty	Amount Charged	Allowed Amount	Copay/ Deduct	Patient Balance	Adjustment	Amt Paid Provider
93015	07/28/10 - 07/28/10	1	325.00	325.00	0.00	65.00	0.00	260.00
	TOTALS		325.00	325.00	0.00	65.00	0.00	260.00

PATIENT: JOHNSON, MARION

PROC CODE	Date of Service From–Thru	Qty	Amount Charged	Allowed Amount	Copay/ Deduct	Patient Balance	Adjustment	Amt Paid Provider
82947	08/18/10 - 08/18/10	1	21.00	21.00	0.00	4.20	0.00	16.80
99215	08/30/10 - 08/30/10	1	135.00	135.00	0.00	27.00	0.00	108.00
93000	08/30/10 - 08/30/10	1	70.00	70.00	0.00	14.00	0.00	56.00
71010	08/30/10 - 08/30/10	1	80.00	80.00	0.00	16.00	0.00	64.00
	TOTALS		306.00	306.00	0.00	61.20	0.00	244.80

PATIENT: SMITH, JAMES

PROC CODE	Date of Service From–Thru	Qty	Amount Charged	Allowed Amount	Copay/ Deduct	Patient Balance	Adjustment	Amt Paid Provider
99212	07/08/10 - 07/08/10	1	44.00	44.00	0.00	8.80	0.00	35.20
99212	08/17/10 - 08/17/10	1	44.00	44.00	0.00	8.80	0.00	35.20
	TOTALS		88.00	88.00	0.00	17.60	0.00	70.40

PAYMENT SUMMARY		TOTAL ALL CLAIMS	
TOTAL AMOUNT PAID	575.20	AMOUNT CHARGED	719.00
PRIOR CREDIT BALANCE	0.00	AMOUNT ALLOWED	719.00
CURRENT CREDIT DEFERRED	0.00	DEDUCTIBLE	0.00
PRIOR CREDIT APPLIED	0.00	COPAY	0.00
NEW CREDIT BALANCE	0.00	OTHER REDUCTION	0.00
NET DISBURSED	575.20	AMOUNT APPROVED	575.20

STATUS CODES:
A - APPROVED   AJ - ADJUSTMENT   IP - IN PROCESS   R - REJECTED   V - VOID

TRICARE
249 Center Street
Columbus, OH 60220

PROVIDER REMITTANCE
THIS IS NOT A BILL
A PAYMENT SUMMARY AND AN EXPLANATION OF
CODES ARE AT THE END OF THIS STATEMENT

FAMILY CARE CENTER
285 STEPHENSON BLVD.
STEPHENSON, OH 60089

Date Prepared:	9/7/10
EFT Number:	7394578
Amount:	$ 200.30

PROVIDER: KATHERINE YAN, M.D.

PATIENT: TANAKA, HIRO

PROC CODE	Date of Service From–Thru	Qty	Amount Charged	Allowed Amount	Copay/ Deduct	Patient Balance	Adjustment	Amt Paid Provider
99212	08/12/10 - 08/12/10	1	44.00	39.60	10.00	0.00	-4.40	29.60
73600	08/12/10 - 08/12/10	1	80.00	72.00	0.00	0.00	-8.00	72.00
99212	08/18/10 - 08/18/10	1	44.00	39.60	10.00	0.00	-4.40	29.60
99212	09/03/10 - 09/03/10	1	44.00	39.60	10.00	0.00	-4.40	29.60
	TOTALS		212.00	190.80	30.00	0.00	-21.20	160.80

PATIENT: PETERSON, ANN

PROC CODE	Date of Service From–Thru	Qty	Amount Charged	Allowed Amount	Copay/ Deduct	Patient Balance	Adjustment	Amt Paid Provider
99201	07/20/10 - 07/20/10	1	55.00	49.50	10.00	0.00	-5.50	39.50
	TOTALS		55.00	49.50	10.00	0.00	-5.50	39.50

PAYMENT SUMMARY		TOTAL ALL CLAIMS	
TOTAL AMOUNT PAID	200.30	AMOUNT CHARGED	267.00
PRIOR CREDIT BALANCE	0.00	AMOUNT ALLOWED	240.30
CURRENT CREDIT DEFERRED	0.00	DEDUCTIBLE	0.00
PRIOR CREDIT APPLIED	0.00	COPAY	40.00
NEW CREDIT BALANCE	0.00	OTHER REDUCTION	0.00
NET DISBURSED	200.30	AMOUNT APPROVED	200.30

STATUS CODES:
A - APPROVED   AJ - ADJUSTMENT   IP - IN PROCESS   R - REJECTED   V - VOID

BLUE CROSS BLUE SHIELD
340 Preston Boulevard
Columbus, OH 60220

PROVIDER REMITTANCE
THIS IS NOT A BILL
A PAYMENT SUMMARY AND AN EXPLANATION OF
CODES ARE AT THE END OF THIS STATEMENT

FAMILY CARE CENTER
285 STEPHENSON BLVD.
STEPHENSON, OH 60089

Date Prepared:	9/7/10
EFT Number:	004567
Amount:	$ 229.60

PROVIDER: KATHERINE YAN, M.D.

PATIENT: LOMOS, CEDERA

PROC CODE	Date of Service From–Thru	Qty	Amount Charged	Allowed Amount	Copay/ Deduct	Patient Balance	Adjustment	Amt Paid Provider
99204	09/03/10 - 09/03/10	1	147.00	147.00	0.00	29.40	0.00	117.60
	TOTALS		147.00	147.00	0.00	29.40	0.00	117.60

PATIENT: LOMOS, LISA

PROC CODE	Date of Service From–Thru	Qty	Amount Charged	Allowed Amount	Copay/ Deduct	Patient Balance	Adjustment	Amt Paid Provider
99383	09/03/10 - 09/03/10	1	140.00	140.00	0.00	28.00	0.00	112.00
	TOTALS		140.00	140.00	0.00	28.00	0.00	112.00

PAYMENT SUMMARY		TOTAL ALL CLAIMS	
TOTAL AMOUNT PAID	229.60	AMOUNT CHARGED	287.00
PRIOR CREDIT BALANCE	0.00	AMOUNT ALLOWED	287.00
CURRENT CREDIT DEFERRED	0.00	DEDUCTIBLE	0.00
PRIOR CREDIT APPLIED	0.00	COPAY	0.00
NEW CREDIT BALANCE	0.00	OTHER REDUCTION	0.00
NET DISBURSED	229.60	AMOUNT APPROVED	229.60

STATUS CODES:
A - APPROVED   AJ - ADJUSTMENT   IP - IN PROCESS   R - REJECTED   V - VOID

BLUE CROSS BLUE SHIELD
340 Preston Boulevard
Columbus, OH 60220

PROVIDER REMITTANCE
THIS IS NOT A BILL
A PAYMENT SUMMARY AND AN EXPLANATION OF
CODES ARE AT THE END OF THIS STATEMENT

FAMILY CARE CENTER
285 STEPHENSON BLVD.
STEPHENSON, OH 60089

Date Prepared:	9/7/10
EFT Number:	3574896
Amount:	$ 52.80

PROVIDER: KATHERINE YAN, M.D.

PATIENT: BARMENSTEIN, ELLEN

PROC CODE	Date of Service From–Thru	Qty	Amount Charged	Allowed Amount	Copay/ Deduct	Patient Balance	Adjustment	Amt Paid Provider
99212	08/28/10 - 08/28/10	1	44.00	44.00	0.00	8.80	0.00	35.20
99211	09/03/10 - 09/03/10	1	30.00	0.00	0.00	30.00***	0.00	0.00
90471	09/03/10 - 09/03/10	1	10.00	10.00	0.00	2.00	0.00	8.00
90658	09/03/10 - 09/03/10	1	12.00	12.00	0.00	2.40	0.00	9.60
	TOTALS		96.00	66.00	0.00	43.20	0.00	52.80

***Not eligible when combined with 90471.

PAYMENT SUMMARY		TOTAL ALL CLAIMS	
TOTAL AMOUNT PAID	52.80	AMOUNT CHARGED	96.00
PRIOR CREDIT BALANCE	0.00	AMOUNT ALLOWED	66.00
CURRENT CREDIT DEFERRED	0.00	DEDUCTIBLE	0.00
PRIOR CREDIT APPLIED	0.00	COPAY	0.00
NEW CREDIT BALANCE	0.00	OTHER REDUCTION	0.00
NET DISBURSED	52.80	AMOUNT APPROVED	52.80

STATUS CODES:
A - APPROVED   AJ - ADJUSTMENT   IP - IN PROCESS   R - REJECTED   V - VOID

ENCOUNTER FORM

10/29/10	1:00pm	Dr. Katherine Yan
DATE	TIME	PROVIDER

Janine Bell		BELJA000
PATIENT NAME		CHART #

OFFICE VISITS - SYMPTOMATIC - NEW		
99201	OF--New Patient Minimal	
99202	OF--New Patient Low	
99203	OF--New Patient Detailed	
99204	OF--New Patient Moderate	
99205	OF--New Patient High	
OFFICE VISITS - SYMPTOMATIC - ESTABLISHED		
99211	OF--Established Patient Minimal	X
99212	OF--Established Patient Low	
99213	OF--Established Patient Detailed	
99214	OF--Established Patient Moderate	
99215	OF--Established Patient High	
PREVENTIVE VISITS - NEW		
99381	Under 1 Year	
99382	1 - 4 Years	
99383	5 - 11 Years	
99384	12 - 17 Years	
99385	18 - 39 Years	
99386	40 - 64 Years	
99387	65 Years & Up	
PREVENTIVE VISITS - ESTABLISHED		
99391	Under 1 Year	
99392	1 - 4 Years	
99393	5 - 11 Years	
99394	12 - 17 Years	
99395	18 - 39 Years	
99396	40 - 64 Years	
99397	65 Years & Up	
PROCEDURES		
12011	Repair of superficial wounds, face	
29125	Short arm splint	
45378	Colonoscopy--diagnostic	
45380	Colonoscopy--biopsy	
71010	Chest x-ray, frontal	
71020	Chest x-ray, frontal and lateral	
73070	Elbow x-ray, AP and lateral	

PROCEDURES		
73090	Forearm x-ray, AP and lateral	
73100	Wrist x-ray, AP and lateral	
73600	Ankle x-ray, AP and lateral	
93000	Electrocardiogram--ECG	
93015	Treadmill stress test	
LABORATORY		
80061	Lipid panel	
82270	Hemoccult--stool screening	
82465	Cholesterol test	
82947	Glucose--quantitative	X
82951	Glucose tolerance test	
83718	HDL cholesterol test	
85007	Manual WBC	
85025	CBC w/diff.	
85651	Erythrocyte sed rate--ESR	
86580	Mantoux test	
87040	Bacterial culture	
87430	Strep screen	
87086	Urine colony count	
87088	Urine culture	
INJECTIONS		
90465	Immunization administration, pt under 8 yrs	
90471	Immunization administration	
90657	Influenza injection, under 35 months	
90658	Influenza injection, older than 3 years	
90703	Tetanus immunization	
90707	MMR immunization	

PB FAMILY CARE CENTER		NOTES
REFERRING PHYSICIAN	NPI	
AUTHORIZATION #		
DIAGNOSIS		
250.00 diabetes mellitus		
PAYMENT AMOUNT		
$15 copayment, check #33		

ENCOUNTER FORM

10/29/10	1:30pm
DATE	TIME

Dr. Katherine Yan
PROVIDER

Felix Suarez
PATIENT NAME

SUAFE000
CHART #

OFFICE VISITS - SYMPTOMATIC - NEW		
99201	OF--New Patient Minimal	
99202	OF--New Patient Low	
99203	OF--New Patient Detailed	
99204	OF--New Patient Moderate	
99205	OF--New Patient High	
OFFICE VISITS - SYMPTOMATIC - ESTABLISHED		
99211	OF--Established Patient Minimal	
99212	OF--Established Patient Low	X
99213	OF--Established Patient Detailed	
99214	OF--Established Patient Moderate	
99215	OF--Established Patient High	
PREVENTIVE VISITS - NEW		
99381	Under 1 Year	
99382	1 - 4 Years	
99383	5 - 11 Years	
99384	12 - 17 Years	
99385	18 - 39 Years	
99386	40 - 64 Years	
99387	65 Years & Up	
PREVENTIVE VISITS - ESTABLISHED		
99391	Under 1 Year	
99392	1 - 4 Years	
99393	5 - 11 Years	
99394	12 - 17 Years	
99395	18 - 39 Years	
99396	40 - 64 Years	
99397	65 Years & Up	
PROCEDURES		
12011	Repair of superficial wounds, face	
29125	Short arm splint	
45378	Colonoscopy--diagnostic	
45380	Colonoscopy--biopsy	
71010	Chest x-ray, frontal	
71020	Chest x-ray, frontal and lateral	
73070	Elbow x-ray, AP and lateral	

PROCEDURES		
73090	Forearm x-ray, AP and lateral	
73100	Wrist x-ray, AP and lateral	
73600	Ankle x-ray, AP and lateral	
93000	Electrocardiogram--ECG	
93015	Treadmill stress test	
LABORATORY		
80061	Lipid panel	
82270	Hemoccult--stool screening	
82465	Cholesterol test	
82947	Glucose--quantitative	
82951	Glucose tolerance test	
83718	HDL cholesterol test	
85007	Manual WBC	
85025	CBC w/diff.	
85651	Erythrocyte sed rate--ESR	
86580	Mantoux test	
87040	Bacterial culture	
87430	Strep screen	
87086	Urine colony count	
87088	Urine culture	
INJECTIONS		
90465	Immunization administration, pt under 8 yrs	
90471	Immunization administration	
90657	Influenza injection, under 35 months	
90658	Influenza injection, older than 3 years	
90703	Tetanus immunization	
90707	MMR immunization	

PB FAMILY CARE CENTER

REFERRING PHYSICIAN

NPI

AUTHORIZATION #

DIAGNOSIS
455.6 hemorrhoids

PAYMENT AMOUNT
$15 copayment, check #3011

NOTES

ENCOUNTER FORM

10/29/10	2:00pm	Dr. Katherine Yan
DATE	TIME	PROVIDER

Sarah Fitzwilliams	FITSA000
PATIENT NAME	CHART #

OFFICE VISITS - SYMPTOMATIC - NEW		
99201	OF--New Patient Minimal	
99202	OF--New Patient Low	
99203	OF--New Patient Detailed	
99204	OF--New Patient Moderate	
99205	OF--New Patient High	
OFFICE VISITS - SYMPTOMATIC - ESTABLISHED		
99211	OF--Established Patient Minimal	X
99212	OF--Established Patient Low	
99213	OF--Established Patient Detailed	
99214	OF--Established Patient Moderate	
99215	OF--Established Patient High	
PREVENTIVE VISITS - NEW		
99381	Under 1 Year	
99382	1 - 4 Years	
99383	5 - 11 Years	
99384	12 - 17 Years	
99385	18 - 39 Years	
99386	40 - 64 Years	
99387	65 Years & Up	
PREVENTIVE VISITS - ESTABLISHED		
99391	Under 1 Year	
99392	1 - 4 Years	
99393	5 - 11 Years	
99394	12 - 17 Years	
99395	18 - 39 Years	
99396	40 - 64 Years	
99397	65 Years & Up	
PROCEDURES		
12011	Repair of superficial wounds, face	
29125	Short arm splint	
45378	Colonoscopy--diagnostic	
45380	Colonoscopy--biopsy	
71010	Chest x-ray, frontal	
71020	Chest x-ray, frontal and lateral	
73070	Elbow x-ray, AP and lateral	

PROCEDURES		
73090	Forearm x-ray, AP and lateral	
73100	Wrist x-ray, AP and lateral	
73600	Ankle x-ray, AP and lateral	
93000	Electrocardiogram--ECG	
93015	Treadmill stress test	
LABORATORY		
80061	Lipid panel	
82270	Hemoccult--stool screening	
82465	Cholesterol test	
82947	Glucose--quantitative	
82951	Glucose tolerance test	
83718	HDL cholesterol test	
85007	Manual WBC	
85025	CBC w/diff.	
85651	Erythrocyte sed rate--ESR	
86580	Mantoux test	
87040	Bacterial culture	
87430	Strep screen	
87086	Urine colony count	
87088	Urine culture	
INJECTIONS		
90465	Immunization administration, pt under 8 yrs	
90471	Immunization administration	
90657	Influenza injection, under 35 months	
90658	Influenza injection, older than 3 years	
90703	Tetanus immunization	
90707	MMR immunization	

PB FAMILY CARE CENTER		NOTES
REFERRING PHYSICIAN	NPI	
AUTHORIZATION #		
DIAGNOSIS 401.9 essential hypertension		
PAYMENT AMOUNT $10 copayment, check #345		

ENCOUNTER FORM

10/29/10	2:30pm	Dr. Katherine Yan
DATE	TIME	PROVIDER

Marion Johnson	JOHMA000
PATIENT NAME	CHART #

OFFICE VISITS - SYMPTOMATIC - NEW		
99201	OF--New Patient Minimal	
99202	OF--New Patient Low	
99203	OF--New Patient Detailed	
99204	OF--New Patient Moderate	
99205	OF--New Patient High	
OFFICE VISITS - SYMPTOMATIC - ESTABLISHED		
99211	OF--Established Patient Minimal	
99212	OF--Established Patient Low	X
99213	OF--Established Patient Detailed	
99214	OF--Established Patient Moderate	
99215	OF--Established Patient High	
PREVENTIVE VISITS - NEW		
99381	Under 1 Year	
99382	1 - 4 Years	
99383	5 - 11 Years	
99384	12 - 17 Years	
99385	18 - 39 Years	
99386	40 - 64 Years	
99387	65 Years & Up	
PREVENTIVE VISITS - ESTABLISHED		
99391	Under 1 Year	
99392	1 - 4 Years	
99393	5 - 11 Years	
99394	12 - 17 Years	
99395	18 - 39 Years	
99396	40 - 64 Years	
99397	65 Years & Up	
PROCEDURES		
12011	Repair of superficial wounds, face	
29125	Short arm splint	
45378	Colonoscopy--diagnostic	
45380	Colonoscopy--biopsy	
71010	Chest x-ray, frontal	X
71020	Chest x-ray, frontal and lateral	
73070	Elbow x-ray, AP and lateral	

PROCEDURES		
73090	Forearm x-ray, AP and lateral	
73100	Wrist x-ray, AP and lateral	
73600	Ankle x-ray, AP and lateral	
93000	Electrocardiogram--ECG	
93015	Treadmill stress test	
LABORATORY		
80061	Lipid panel	
82270	Hemoccult--stool screening	
82465	Cholesterol test	
82947	Glucose--quantitative	
82951	Glucose tolerance test	
83718	HDL cholesterol test	
85007	Manual WBC	
85025	CBC w/diff.	
85651	Erythrocyte sed rate--ESR	
86580	Mantoux test	
87040	Bacterial culture	
87430	Strep screen	X
87086	Urine colony count	
87088	Urine culture	
INJECTIONS		
90465	Immunization administration, pt under 8 yrs	
90471	Immunization administration	
90657	Influenza injection, under 35 months	
90658	Influenza injection, older than 3 years	
90703	Tetanus immunization	
90707	MMR immunization	

PB FAMILY CARE CENTER		NOTES
REFERRING PHYSICIAN	NPI	
AUTHORIZATION #		
DIAGNOSIS 490 bronchitis, unqualified		
PAYMENT AMOUNT		

PATIENT INFORMATION FORM

THIS SECTION REFERS TO PATIENT ONLY

Name: Darla Andrews	Sex: F	Marital Status: ☐S ☒M ☐D ☐W	Birth Date: 6/8/78

Address: 1 West 8th Street

SS#: 332-49-0432

City: Stephenson	State: OH	Zip: 60089

Employer: Western Drug (full-time)

Home Phone: 614-241-3321

Employer's Address:

Work Phone: 614-721-0032

City: State: Zip:

Spouse's Name:

Spouse's Employer:

Emergency Contact:

Relationship: Phone #:

FILL IN IF PATIENT IS A MINOR

Parent/Guardian's Name:	Sex:	Marital Status: ☐S ☐M ☐D ☐W	Birth Date:

Phone:

SS#:

Address:

Employer:

City:	State:	Zip:

Employer's Address:

Student Status:

City: State: Zip:

INSURANCE INFORMATION

Primary Insurance Company: Physician's Choice

Secondary Insurance Company:

Subscriber's Name: (same)	Birth Date: 6/8/78

Subscriber's Name: Birth Date:

Plan:	SS#: 332-49-0432

Plan:

Policy #: 1122191	Group #: 83

Policy #:   Group #:

Copayment: $15	Deductible:	Price Code: A

OTHER INFORMATION

Reason for visit: Chest pain

Allergy to Medication (list):

Name of referring physician:

If auto accident, list date and state in which it occurred:

I authorize treatment and agree to pay all fees and charges for the person named above. I agree to pay all charges shown by statements, promptly upon their presentation, unless credit arrangements are agreed upon in writing.

I authorize payment directly to FAMILY CARE CENTER of insurance benefits otherwise payable to me. I hereby authorize the release of any medical information necessary in order to process a claim for payment in my behalf.

Darla Andrews	11/1/10
(Patient's Signature/Parent or Guardian's Signature)	(Date)

I plan to make payment of my medical expenses as follows (check one or more):

  X Insurance (as above)   X Cash/Check/Credit/Debit Card _____ Medicare _____ Medicaid _____ Workers' Comp.

PATIENT INFORMATION FORM

THIS SECTION REFERS TO PATIENT ONLY

Name: William Andrews	Sex: M	Marital Status: ☐ S ☒ M ☐ D ☐ W	Birth Date: 12/1/75

Address: 1 West 8th Street	SS#: 341-59-9392

City: Stephenson	State: OH	Zip: 60089	Employer: Wheeler, Sampson, Hull (full-time)

Home Phone: 614-241-3321	Employer's Address:

Work Phone: 614-836-8579	City:	State:	Zip:

Spouse's Name:	Spouse's Employer:

Emergency Contact:	Relationship:	Phone #:

FILL IN IF PATIENT IS A MINOR

Parent/Guardian's Name:	Sex:	Marital Status: ☐ S ☐ M ☐ D ☐ W	Birth Date:

Phone:	SS#:

Address:	Employer:

City:	State:	Zip:	Employer's Address:

Student Status:	City:	State:	Zip:

INSURANCE INFORMATION

Primary Insurance Company: Physician's Choice	Secondary Insurance Company:

Subscriber's Name: Darla Andrews	Birth Date: 6/8/78	Subscriber's Name:	Birth Date:

Plan:	SS#: 332-49-0432	Plan:

Policy #: 1122191	Group #: 83	Policy #:	Group #:

Copayment: $15	Deductible:	Price Code: A

OTHER INFORMATION

Reason for visit: Routine physical	Allergy to Medication (list): Penicillin

Name of referring physician:	If auto accident, list date and state in which it occurred:

I authorize treatment and agree to pay all fees and charges for the person named above. I agree to pay all charges shown by statements, promptly upon their presentation, unless credit arrangements are agreed upon in writing.

I authorize payment directly to FAMILY CARE CENTER of insurance benefits otherwise payable to me. I hereby authorize the release of any medical information necessary in order to process a claim for payment in my behalf.

William Andrews	11/1/10
(Patient's Signature/Parent or Guardian's Signature)	(Date)

I plan to make payment of my medical expenses as follows (check one or more):

__X__ Insurance (as above)   __X__ Cash/Check/Credit/Debit Card   _____ Medicare   _____ Medicaid   _____ Workers' Comp.

ENCOUNTER FORM

11/1/10	**9:00am**
DATE	TIME

Dr. Katherine Yan
PROVIDER

Darla Andrews
PATIENT NAME

ANDDA000
CHART #

OFFICE VISITS - SYMPTOMATIC - NEW		
99201	OF--New Patient Minimal	
99202	OF--New Patient Low	
99203	OF--New Patient Detailed	X
99204	OF--New Patient Moderate	
99205	OF--New Patient High	
OFFICE VISITS - SYMPTOMATIC - ESTABLISHED		
99211	OF--Established Patient Minimal	
99212	OF--Established Patient Low	
99213	OF--Established Patient Detailed	
99214	OF--Established Patient Moderate	
99215	OF--Established Patient High	
PREVENTIVE VISITS - NEW		
99381	Under 1 Year	
99382	1 - 4 Years	
99383	5 - 11 Years	
99384	12 - 17 Years	
99385	18 - 39 Years	
99386	40 - 64 Years	
99387	65 Years & Up	
PREVENTIVE VISITS - ESTABLISHED		
99391	Under 1 Year	
99392	1 - 4 Years	
99393	5 - 11 Years	
99394	12 - 17 Years	
99395	18 - 39 Years	
99396	40 - 64 Years	
99397	65 Years & Up	
PROCEDURES		
12011	Repair of superficial wounds, face	
29125	Short arm splint	
45378	Colonoscopy--diagnostic	
45380	Colonoscopy--biopsy	
71010	Chest x-ray, frontal	X
71020	Chest x-ray, frontal and lateral	
73070	Elbow x-ray, AP and lateral	

PROCEDURES		
73090	Forearm x-ray, AP and lateral	
73100	Wrist x-ray, AP and lateral	
73600	Ankle x-ray, AP and lateral	
93000	Electrocardiogram--ECG	X
93015	Treadmill stress test	
LABORATORY		
80061	Lipid panel	
82270	Hemoccult--stool screening	
82465	Cholesterol test	
82947	Glucose--quantitative	
82951	Glucose tolerance test	
83718	HDL cholesterol test	
85007	Manual WBC	
85025	CBC w/diff.	
85651	Erythrocyte sed rate--ESR	
86580	Mantoux test	
87040	Bacterial culture	
87430	Strep screen	
87086	Urine colony count	
87088	Urine culture	
INJECTIONS		
90465	Immunization administration, pt under 8 yrs	
90471	Immunization administration	
90657	Influenza injection, under 35 months	
90658	Influenza injection, older than 3 years	
90703	Tetanus immunization	
90707	MMR immunization	

PB FAMILY CARE CENTER		NOTES
REFERRING PHYSICIAN	NPI	
AUTHORIZATION #		
DIAGNOSIS		
786.50 chest pain		
PAYMENT AMOUNT		
$15 copayment, check #123		

ENCOUNTER FORM

11/1/10	9:30am	Dr. Katherine Yan
DATE	TIME	PROVIDER

William Andrews		ANDWI000
PATIENT NAME		CHART #

OFFICE VISITS - SYMPTOMATIC - NEW		
99201	OF--New Patient Minimal	
99202	OF--New Patient Low	
99203	OF--New Patient Detailed	
99204	OF--New Patient Moderate	
99205	OF--New Patient High	
OFFICE VISITS - SYMPTOMATIC - ESTABLISHED		
99211	OF--Established Patient Minimal	
99212	OF--Established Patient Low	
99213	OF--Established Patient Detailed	
99214	OF--Established Patient Moderate	
99215	OF--Established Patient High	
PREVENTIVE VISITS - NEW		
99381	Under 1 Year	
99382	1 - 4 Years	
99383	5 - 11 Years	
99384	12 - 17 Years	
99385	18 - 39 Years	X
99386	40 - 64 Years	
99387	65 Years & Up	
PREVENTIVE VISITS - ESTABLISHED		
99391	Under 1 Year	
99392	1 - 4 Years	
99393	5 - 11 Years	
99394	12 - 17 Years	
99395	18 - 39 Years	
99396	40 - 64 Years	
99397	65 Years & Up	
PROCEDURES		
12011	Repair of superficial wounds, face	
29125	Short arm splint	
45378	Colonoscopy--diagnostic	
45380	Colonoscopy--biopsy	
71010	Chest x-ray, frontal	
71020	Chest x-ray, frontal and lateral	
73070	Elbow x-ray, AP and lateral	

PROCEDURES		
73090	Forearm x-ray, AP and lateral	
73100	Wrist x-ray, AP and lateral	
73600	Ankle x-ray, AP and lateral	
93000	Electrocardiogram--ECG	
93015	Treadmill stress test	
LABORATORY		
80061	Lipid panel	
82270	Hemoccult--stool screening	
82465	Cholesterol test	
82947	Glucose--quantitative	
82951	Glucose tolerance test	
83718	HDL cholesterol test	
85007	Manual WBC	
85025	CBC w/diff.	
85651	Erythrocyte sed rate--ESR	
86580	Mantoux test	
87040	Bacterial culture	
87430	Strep screen	
87086	Urine colony count	
87088	Urine culture	
INJECTIONS		
90465	Immunization administration, pt under 8 yrs	
90471	Immunization administration	
90657	Influenza injection, under 35 months	
90658	Influenza injection, older than 3 years	
90703	Tetanus immunization	
90707	MMR immunization	

PB FAMILY CARE CENTER		NOTES
REFERRING PHYSICIAN	NPI	
AUTHORIZATION #		
DIAGNOSIS		
v70.0 preventive physical exam		
PAYMENT AMOUNT		
$15 copayment, check #124		

ENCOUNTER FORM

11/1/10	**10:00am**	**Dr. Katherine Yan**	
DATE	TIME	PROVIDER	
Cedera Lomos		**LOMCE000**	
PATIENT NAME		CHART #	

OFFICE VISITS - SYMPTOMATIC - NEW		
99201	OF--New Patient Minimal	
99202	OF--New Patient Low	
99203	OF--New Patient Detailed	
99204	OF--New Patient Moderate	
99205	OF--New Patient High	
OFFICE VISITS - SYMPTOMATIC - ESTABLISHED		
99211	OF--Established Patient Minimal	X
99212	OF--Established Patient Low	
99213	OF--Established Patient Detailed	
99214	OF--Established Patient Moderate	
99215	OF--Established Patient High	
PREVENTIVE VISITS - NEW		
99381	Under 1 Year	
99382	1 - 4 Years	
99383	5 - 11 Years	
99384	12 - 17 Years	
99385	18 - 39 Years	
99386	40 - 64 Years	
99387	65 Years & Up	
PREVENTIVE VISITS - ESTABLISHED		
99391	Under 1 Year	
99392	1 - 4 Years	
99393	5 - 11 Years	
99394	12 - 17 Years	
99395	18 - 39 Years	
99396	40 - 64 Years	
99397	65 Years & Up	
PROCEDURES		
12011	Repair of superficial wounds, face	
29125	Short arm splint	
45378	Colonoscopy--diagnostic	
45380	Colonoscopy--biopsy	
71010	Chest x-ray, frontal	
71020	Chest x-ray, frontal and lateral	
73070	Elbow x-ray, AP and lateral	

PROCEDURES		
73090	Forearm x-ray, AP and lateral	
73100	Wrist x-ray, AP and lateral	
73600	Ankle x-ray, AP and lateral	
93000	Electrocardiogram--ECG	
93015	Treadmill stress test	
LABORATORY		
80061	Lipid panel	
82270	Hemoccult--stool screening	
82465	Cholesterol test	
82947	Glucose--quantitative	
82951	Glucose tolerance test	
83718	HDL cholesterol test	
85007	Manual WBC	
85025	CBC w/diff.	
85651	Erythrocyte sed rate--ESR	
86580	Mantoux test	
87040	Bacterial culture	
87430	Strep screen	
87086	Urine colony count	
87088	Urine culture	
INJECTIONS		
90465	Immunization administration, pt under 8 yrs	
90471	Immunization administration	
90657	Influenza injection, under 35 months	
90658	Influenza injection, older than 3 years	
90703	Tetanus immunization	
90707	MMR immunization	

PB FAMILY CARE CENTER		NOTES
REFERRING PHYSICIAN	NPI	
AUTHORIZATION #		
DIAGNOSIS		
473.9 Chronic sinusitis		
PAYMENT AMOUNT		

ENCOUNTER FORM

11/1/10	**10:30am**
DATE	TIME

Dr. Katherine Yan
PROVIDER

Stanley Feldman
PATIENT NAME

FELST000
CHART #

OFFICE VISITS - SYMPTOMATIC - NEW		
99201	OF--New Patient Minimal	
99202	OF--New Patient Low	
99203	OF--New Patient Detailed	
99204	OF--New Patient Moderate	
99205	OF--New Patient High	
OFFICE VISITS - SYMPTOMATIC - ESTABLISHED		
99211	OF--Established Patient Minimal	X
99212	OF--Established Patient Low	
99213	OF--Established Patient Detailed	
99214	OF--Established Patient Moderate	
99215	OF--Established Patient High	
PREVENTIVE VISITS - NEW		
99381	Under 1 Year	
99382	1 - 4 Years	
99383	5 - 11 Years	
99384	12 - 17 Years	
99385	18 - 39 Years	
99386	40 - 64 Years	
99387	65 Years & Up	
PREVENTIVE VISITS - ESTABLISHED		
99391	Under 1 Year	
99392	1 - 4 Years	
99393	5 - 11 Years	
99394	12 - 17 Years	
99395	18 - 39 Years	
99396	40 - 64 Years	
99397	65 Years & Up	
PROCEDURES		
12011	Repair of superficial wounds, face	
29125	Short arm splint	
45378	Colonoscopy--diagnostic	
45380	Colonoscopy--biopsy	
71010	Chest x-ray, frontal	
71020	Chest x-ray, frontal and lateral	
73070	Elbow x-ray, AP and lateral	

PROCEDURES		
73090	Forearm x-ray, AP and lateral	
73100	Wrist x-ray, AP and lateral	
73600	Ankle x-ray, AP and lateral	
93000	Electrocardiogram--ECG	
93015	Treadmill stress test	
LABORATORY		
80061	Lipid panel	X
82270	Hemoccult--stool screening	
82465	Cholesterol test	
82947	Glucose--quantitative	
82951	Glucose tolerance test	
83718	HDL cholesterol test	
85007	Manual WBC	
85025	CBC w/diff.	
85651	Erythrocyte sed rate--ESR	
86580	Mantoux test	
87040	Bacterial culture	
87430	Strep screen	
87086	Urine colony count	
87088	Urine culture	
INJECTIONS		
90465	Immunization administration, pt under 8 yrs	
90471	Immunization administration	
90657	Influenza injection, under 35 months	
90658	Influenza injection, older than 3 years	
90703	Tetanus immunization	
90707	MMR immunization	

PB FAMILY CARE CENTER

REFERRING PHYSICIAN	NPI
AUTHORIZATION #	

DIAGNOSIS

272.0 hypercholesterolemia

PAYMENT AMOUNT

NOTES

ENCOUNTER FORM

11/1/10	1:45pm	Dr. Katherine Yan
DATE	TIME	PROVIDER

Ethan Sampson	SAMET000
PATIENT NAME	CHART #

OFFICE VISITS - SYMPTOMATIC - NEW		
99201	OF--New Patient Minimal	
99202	OF--New Patient Low	
99203	OF--New Patient Detailed	
99204	OF--New Patient Moderate	
99205	OF--New Patient High	
OFFICE VISITS - SYMPTOMATIC - ESTABLISHED		
99211	OF--Established Patient Minimal	
99212	OF--Established Patient Low	
99213	OF--Established Patient Detailed	
99214	OF--Established Patient Moderate	X
99215	OF--Established Patient High	
PREVENTIVE VISITS - NEW		
99381	Under 1 Year	
99382	1 - 4 Years	
99383	5 - 11 Years	
99384	12 - 17 Years	
99385	18 - 39 Years	
99386	40 - 64 Years	
99387	65 Years & Up	
PREVENTIVE VISITS - ESTABLISHED		
99391	Under 1 Year	
99392	1 - 4 Years	
99393	5 - 11 Years	
99394	12 - 17 Years	
99395	18 - 39 Years	
99396	40 - 64 Years	
99397	65 Years & Up	
PROCEDURES		
12011	Repair of superficial wounds, face	
29125	Short arm splint	
45378	Colonoscopy--diagnostic	
45380	Colonoscopy--biopsy	
71010	Chest x-ray, frontal	
71020	Chest x-ray, frontal and lateral	
73070	Elbow x-ray, AP and lateral	

PROCEDURES		
73090	Forearm x-ray, AP and lateral	X
73100	Wrist x-ray, AP and lateral	
73600	Ankle x-ray, AP and lateral	
93000	Electrocardiogram--ECG	
93015	Treadmill stress test	
LABORATORY		
80061	Lipid panel	
82270	Hemoccult--stool screening	
82465	Cholesterol test	
82947	Glucose--quantitative	
82951	Glucose tolerance test	
83718	HDL cholesterol test	
85007	Manual WBC	
85025	CBC w/diff.	
85651	Erythrocyte sed rate--ESR	
86580	Mantoux test	
87040	Bacterial culture	
87430	Strep screen	
87086	Urine colony count	
87088	Urine culture	
INJECTIONS		
90465	Immunization administration, pt under 8 yrs	
90471	Immunization administration	
90657	Influenza injection, under 35 months	
90658	Influenza injection, older than 3 years	
90703	Tetanus immunization	
90707	MMR immunization	

PB FAMILY CARE CENTER

REFERRING PHYSICIAN	NPI

NOTES

AUTHORIZATION #

DIAGNOSIS
848.9 sprain or strain

PAYMENT AMOUNT
$15 copayment, check #129

PATIENT INFORMATION FORM

THIS SECTION REFERS TO PATIENT ONLY

Name: Jo Black	Sex: F	Marital Status: ☒ S ☐ M ☐ D ☐ W	Birth Date: 1/11/58

Address: 3 Parkway Road	SS#: 321-22-8787

City: Stephenson	State: OH	Zip: 60089	Employer: Barden Elementary School (full-time)

Home Phone: 614-555-8989	Employer's Address:

Work Phone: 614-879-2000	City:	State:	Zip:

Spouse's Name:	Spouse's Employer:

Emergency Contact:	Relationship:	Phone #:

FILL IN IF PATIENT IS A MINOR

Parent/Guardian's Name:	Sex:	Marital Status: ☐ S ☐ M ☐ D ☐ W	Birth Date:

Phone:	SS#:

Address:	Employer:

City:	State:	Zip:	Employer's Address:

Student Status:	City:	State:	Zip:

INSURANCE INFORMATION

Primary Insurance Company: Blue Cross/Blue Shield	Secondary Insurance Company:

Subscriber's Name: (same)	Birth Date: 1/11/58	Subscriber's Name:	Birth Date:

Plan:	SS#: 321-22-8787	Plan:

Policy #: 321228787	Group #: BE134	Policy #:	Group #:

Copayment:	Deductible: $200	Price Code: A

OTHER INFORMATION

Reason for visit:	Allergy to Medication (list):

Name of referring physician:	If auto accident, list date and state in which it occurred:

I authorize treatment and agree to pay all fees and charges for the person named above. I agree to pay all charges shown by statements, promptly upon their presentation, unless credit arrangements are agreed upon in writing.

I authorize payment directly to FAMILY CARE CENTER of insurance benefits otherwise payable to me. I hereby authorize the release of any medical information necessary in order to process a claim for payment in my behalf.

Jo Black	11/1/10
(Patient's Signature/Parent or Guardian's Signature)	(Date)

I plan to make payment of my medical expenses as follows (check one or more):

__X__ Insurance (as above)   __X__ Cash/Check/Credit/Debit Card   _____ Medicare   _____ Medicaid   _____ Workers' Comp.

ENCOUNTER FORM

11/1/10	**2:00pm**	**Dr. Katherine Yan**
DATE	TIME	PROVIDER
Jo Black		**BLAJO000**
PATIENT NAME		CHART #

OFFICE VISITS - SYMPTOMATIC - NEW		
99201	OF--New Patient Minimal	
99202	OF--New Patient Low	
99203	OF--New Patient Detailed	X
99204	OF--New Patient Moderate	
99205	OF--New Patient High	
OFFICE VISITS - SYMPTOMATIC - ESTABLISHED		
99211	OF--Established Patient Minimal	
99212	OF--Established Patient Low	
99213	OF--Established Patient Detailed	
99214	OF--Established Patient Moderate	
99215	OF--Established Patient High	
PREVENTIVE VISITS - NEW		
99381	Under 1 Year	
99382	1 - 4 Years	
99383	5 - 11 Years	
99384	12 - 17 Years	
99385	18 - 39 Years	
99386	40 - 64 Years	
99387	65 Years & Up	
PREVENTIVE VISITS - ESTABLISHED		
99391	Under 1 Year	
99392	1 - 4 Years	
99393	5 - 11 Years	
99394	12 - 17 Years	
99395	18 - 39 Years	
99396	40 - 64 Years	
99397	65 Years & Up	
PROCEDURES		
12011	Repair of superficial wounds, face	
29125	Short arm splint	
45378	Colonoscopy--diagnostic	
45380	Colonoscopy--biopsy	
71010	Chest x-ray, frontal	
71020	Chest x-ray, frontal and lateral	
73070	Elbow x-ray, AP and lateral	

PROCEDURES		
73090	Forearm x-ray, AP and lateral	
73100	Wrist x-ray, AP and lateral	
73600	Ankle x-ray, AP and lateral	
93000	Electrocardiogram--ECG	X
93015	Treadmill stress test	
LABORATORY		
80061	Lipid panel	
82270	Hemoccult--stool screening	
82465	Cholesterol test	
82947	Glucose--quantitative	
82951	Glucose tolerance test	
83718	HDL cholesterol test	
85007	Manual WBC	
85025	CBC w/diff.	
85651	Erythrocyte sed rate--ESR	
86580	Mantoux test	
87040	Bacterial culture	
87430	Strep screen	
87086	Urine colony count	
87088	Urine culture	
INJECTIONS		
90465	Immunization administration, pt under 8 yrs	
90471	Immunization administration	
90657	Influenza injection, under 35 months	
90658	Influenza injection, older than 3 years	
90703	Tetanus immunization	
90707	MMR immunization	

PB FAMILY CARE CENTER		NOTES
REFERRING PHYSICIAN	NPI	
AUTHORIZATION #		
DIAGNOSIS		
427.9 Arrhythmia		
PAYMENT AMOUNT		

ENCOUNTER FORM

11/1/10	2:30pm		Dr. Katherine Yan
DATE	TIME		PROVIDER

Sarina Bell		BELSA001
PATIENT NAME		CHART #

OFFICE VISITS - SYMPTOMATIC - NEW		
99201	OF--New Patient Minimal	
99202	OF--New Patient Low	
99203	OF--New Patient Detailed	
99204	OF--New Patient Moderate	
99205	OF--New Patient High	

OFFICE VISITS - SYMPTOMATIC - ESTABLISHED		
99211	OF--Established Patient Minimal	
99212	OF--Established Patient Low	X
99213	OF--Established Patient Detailed	
99214	OF--Established Patient Moderate	
99215	OF--Established Patient High	

PREVENTIVE VISITS - NEW		
99381	Under 1 Year	
99382	1 - 4 Years	
99383	5 - 11 Years	
99384	12 - 17 Years	
99385	18 - 39 Years	
99386	40 - 64 Years	
99387	65 Years & Up	

PREVENTIVE VISITS - ESTABLISHED		
99391	Under 1 Year	
99392	1 - 4 Years	
99393	5 - 11 Years	
99394	12 - 17 Years	
99395	18 - 39 Years	
99396	40 - 64 Years	
99397	65 Years & Up	

PROCEDURES		
12011	Repair of superficial wounds, face	X
29125	Short arm splint	
45378	Colonoscopy--diagnostic	
45380	Colonoscopy--biopsy	
71010	Chest x-ray, frontal	
71020	Chest x-ray, frontal and lateral	
73070	Elbow x-ray, AP and lateral	

PROCEDURES		
73090	Forearm x-ray, AP and lateral	
73100	Wrist x-ray, AP and lateral	
73600	Ankle x-ray, AP and lateral	
93000	Electrocardiogram--ECG	
93015	Treadmill stress test	

LABORATORY		
80061	Lipid panel	
82270	Hemoccult--stool screening	
82465	Cholesterol test	
82947	Glucose--quantitative	
82951	Glucose tolerance test	
83718	HDL cholesterol test	
85007	Manual WBC	
85025	CBC w/diff.	
85651	Erythrocyte sed rate--ESR	
86580	Mantoux test	
87040	Bacterial culture	
87430	Strep screen	
87086	Urine colony count	
87088	Urine culture	

INJECTIONS		
90465	Immunization administration, pt under 8 yrs	
90471	Immunization administration	
90657	Influenza injection, under 35 months	
90658	Influenza injection, older than 3 years	
90703	Tetanus immunization	
90707	MMR immunization	

PB FAMILY CARE CENTER		NOTES
REFERRING PHYSICIAN	NPI	
AUTHORIZATION #		
DIAGNOSIS 870.0 laceration of eyelid		
PAYMENT AMOUNT $15 copayment, check #1421		

U.S. Life
2788 Broadway
New York, NY 10021

PROVIDER REMITTANCE
THIS IS NOT A BILL
A PAYMENT SUMMARY AND AN EXPLANATION OF
CODES ARE AT THE END OF THIS STATEMENT

FAMILY CARE CENTER
285 STEPHENSON BLVD.
STEPHENSON, OH 60089

Date Prepared:	11/1/10
EFT Number:	34698
Amount:	$ 55.50

PROVIDER: KATHERINE YAN, M.D.

PATIENT: BELL, JANINE

PROC CODE	Date of Service From–Thru	Qty	Amount Charged	Allowed Amount	Copay/ Deduct	Patient Balance	Adjustment	Amt Paid Provider
99211	10/29/10 - 10/29/10	1	30.00	27.00	15.00	0.00	-3.00	12.00
82947	10/29/10 - 10/29/10	1	21.00	18.90	0.00	0.00	-2.10	18.90
	TOTALS		51.00	45.90	15.00	0.00	-5.10	30.90

PATIENT: SUAREZ, FELIX

PROC CODE	Date of Service From–Thru	Qty	Amount Charged	Allowed Amount	Copay/ Deduct	Patient Balance	Adjustment	Amt Paid Provider
99212	10/29/10 - 10/29/10	1	44.00	39.60	15.00	0.00	-4.40	24.60
	TOTALS		44.00	39.60	15.00	0.00	-4.40	24.60

PAYMENT SUMMARY		TOTAL ALL CLAIMS	
TOTAL AMOUNT PAID	55.50	AMOUNT CHARGED	95.00
PRIOR CREDIT BALANCE	0.00	AMOUNT ALLOWED	85.50
CURRENT CREDIT DEFERRED	0.00	DEDUCTIBLE	0.00
PRIOR CREDIT APPLIED	0.00	COPAY	30.00
NEW CREDIT BALANCE	0.00	OTHER REDUCTION	0.00
NET DISBURSED	55.50	AMOUNT APPROVED	55.50

STATUS CODES:
A - APPROVED   AJ - ADJUSTMENT   IP - IN PROCESS   R - REJECTED   V - VOID

ENCOUNTER FORM

11/3/10	9:00am
DATE	TIME

John Gardiner
PATIENT NAME

Dr. Katherine Yan
PROVIDER

GARJO000
CHART #

OFFICE VISITS - SYMPTOMATIC - NEW		
99201	OF--New Patient Minimal	
99202	OF--New Patient Low	
99203	OF--New Patient Detailed	
99204	OF--New Patient Moderate	
99205	OF--New Patient High	

OFFICE VISITS - SYMPTOMATIC - ESTABLISHED		
99211	OF--Established Patient Minimal	X
99212	OF--Established Patient Low	
99213	OF--Established Patient Detailed	
99214	OF--Established Patient Moderate	
99215	OF--Established Patient High	

PREVENTIVE VISITS - NEW		
99381	Under 1 Year	
99382	1 - 4 Years	
99383	5 - 11 Years	
99384	12 - 17 Years	
99385	18 - 39 Years	
99386	40 - 64 Years	
99387	65 Years & Up	

PREVENTIVE VISITS - ESTABLISHED		
99391	Under 1 Year	
99392	1 - 4 Years	
99393	5 - 11 Years	
99394	12 - 17 Years	
99395	18 - 39 Years	
99396	40 - 64 Years	
99397	65 Years & Up	

PROCEDURES		
12011	Repair of superficial wounds, face	
29125	Short arm splint	
45378	Colonoscopy--diagnostic	
45380	Colonoscopy--biopsy	
71010	Chest x-ray, frontal	
71020	Chest x-ray, frontal and lateral	
73070	Elbow x-ray, AP and lateral	

PROCEDURES		
73090	Forearm x-ray, AP and lateral	
73100	Wrist x-ray, AP and lateral	
73600	Ankle x-ray, AP and lateral	
93000	Electrocardiogram--ECG	
93015	Treadmill stress test	

LABORATORY		
80061	Lipid panel	
82270	Hemoccult--stool screening	
82465	Cholesterol test	
82947	Glucose--quantitative	
82951	Glucose tolerance test	
83718	HDL cholesterol test	
85007	Manual WBC	
85025	CBC w/diff.	
85651	Erythrocyte sed rate--ESR	
86580	Mantoux test	
87040	Bacterial culture	
87430	Strep screen	
87086	Urine colony count	
87088	Urine culture	

INJECTIONS		
90465	Immunization administration, pt under 8 yrs	
90471	Immunization administration	
90657	Influenza injection, under 35 months	
90658	Influenza injection, older than 3 years	
90703	Tetanus immunization	
90707	MMR immunization	

PB FAMILY CARE CENTER		NOTES
REFERRING PHYSICIAN	NPI	
AUTHORIZATION #		
DIAGNOSIS 487.1 influenza		
PAYMENT AMOUNT $15 copayment, check #2327		

Family Care Center
285 Stephenson Boulevard
Stephenson, OH 60089
614-555-0100

Things to Do Today

Date _____11/3/2010_____

Patient _____Paul Ramos_____

_____

Paul Ramos has a new home telephone number: _____

_____

614-332-4398 _____

PATIENT INFORMATION FORM

THIS SECTION REFERS TO PATIENT ONLY

| Name: Sam Wu | Sex: M | Marital Status: ☐ S ☐ M ☒ D ☐ W | Birth Date: 8/8/52 |

Address: 4701 Plymouth Avenue

SS#: 381-77-9138

| City: Stephenson | State: OH | Zip: 60089 | Employer: Stephenson Construction (full-time) |

Home Phone: 614-931-3319

Employer's Address:

Work Phone: 614-555-3211

City: State: Zip:

Spouse's Name:

Spouse's Employer:

Emergency Contact:

Relationship: Phone #:

FILL IN IF PATIENT IS A MINOR

| Parent/Guardian's Name: | Sex: | Marital Status: ☐ S ☐ M ☐ D ☐ W | Birth Date: |

Phone:

SS#:

Address:

Employer:

City: State: Zip:

Employer's Address:

Student Status:

City: State: Zip:

INSURANCE INFORMATION

Primary Insurance Company: U.S. Life

Secondary Insurance Company:

| Subscriber's Name: (same) | Birth Date: 8/8/52 | Subscriber's Name: | Birth Date: |

| Plan: | SS#: 381-77-9138 | Plan: |

| Policy #: 381779138 | Group #: 931 | Policy #: | Group #: |

| Copayment: $15 | Deductible: | Price Code: A |

OTHER INFORMATION

Reason for visit: Sprained arm

Allergy to Medication (list):

Name of referring physician:

If auto accident, list date and state in which it occurred: 10/31/10, OH

I authorize treatment and agree to pay all fees and charges for the person named above. I agree to pay all charges shown by statements, promptly upon their presentation, unless credit arrangements are agreed upon in writing.

I authorize payment directly to FAMILY CARE CENTER of insurance benefits otherwise payable to me. I hereby authorize the release of any medical information necessary in order to process a claim for payment in my behalf.

| Sam Wu | 11/3/10 |
| (Patient's Signature/Parent or Guardian's Signature) | (Date) |

I plan to make payment of my medical expenses as follows (check one or more):

__X__ Insurance (as above)   __X__ Cash/Check/Credit/Debit Card   _____ Medicare   _____ Medicaid   _____ Workers' Comp.

ENCOUNTER FORM

11/3/10	**9:30am**
DATE	TIME

Dr. Katherine Yan
PROVIDER

Sam Wu
PATIENT NAME

WUSA0000
CHART #

OFFICE VISITS - SYMPTOMATIC - NEW		
99201	OF--New Patient Minimal	
99202	OF--New Patient Low	X
99203	OF--New Patient Detailed	
99204	OF--New Patient Moderate	
99205	OF--New Patient High	
OFFICE VISITS - SYMPTOMATIC - ESTABLISHED		
99211	OF--Established Patient Minimal	
99212	OF--Established Patient Low	
99213	OF--Established Patient Detailed	
99214	OF--Established Patient Moderate	
99215	OF--Established Patient High	
PREVENTIVE VISITS - NEW		
99381	Under 1 Year	
99382	1 - 4 Years	
99383	5 - 11 Years	
99384	12 - 17 Years	
99385	18 - 39 Years	
99386	40 - 64 Years	
99387	65 Years & Up	
PREVENTIVE VISITS - ESTABLISHED		
99391	Under 1 Year	
99392	1 - 4 Years	
99393	5 - 11 Years	
99394	12 - 17 Years	
99395	18 - 39 Years	
99396	40 - 64 Years	
99397	65 Years & Up	
PROCEDURES		
12011	Repair of superficial wounds, face	
29125	Short arm splint	
45378	Colonoscopy--diagnostic	
45380	Colonoscopy--biopsy	
71010	Chest x-ray, frontal	
71020	Chest x-ray, frontal and lateral	
73070	Elbow x-ray, AP and lateral	X

PROCEDURES		
73090	Forearm x-ray, AP and lateral	X
73100	Wrist x-ray, AP and lateral	
73600	Ankle x-ray, AP and lateral	
93000	Electrocardiogram--ECG	
93015	Treadmill stress test	
LABORATORY		
80061	Lipid panel	
82270	Hemoccult--stool screening	
82465	Cholesterol test	
82947	Glucose--quantitative	
82951	Glucose tolerance test	
83718	HDL cholesterol test	
85007	Manual WBC	
85025	CBC w/diff.	
85651	Erythrocyte sed rate--ESR	
86580	Mantoux test	
87040	Bacterial culture	
87430	Strep screen	
87086	Urine colony count	
87088	Urine culture	
INJECTIONS		
90465	Immunization administration, pt under 8 yrs	
90471	Immunization administration	
90657	Influenza injection, under 35 months	
90658	Influenza injection, older than 3 years	
90703	Tetanus immunization	
90707	MMR immunization	

PB FAMILY CARE CENTER		NOTES
REFERRING PHYSICIAN	NPI	
AUTHORIZATION #		
DIAGNOSIS 848.9 sprain		
PAYMENT AMOUNT $15 copayment, check #561		

ENCOUNTER FORM

11/3/10	10:00am
DATE	TIME

Paul Ramos
PATIENT NAME

Dr. Katherine Yan
PROVIDER

RAMPA000
CHART #

OFFICE VISITS - SYMPTOMATIC - NEW		
99201	OF--New Patient Minimal	
99202	OF--New Patient Low	
99203	OF--New Patient Detailed	
99204	OF--New Patient Moderate	
99205	OF--New Patient High	
OFFICE VISITS - SYMPTOMATIC - ESTABLISHED		
99211	OF--Established Patient Minimal	
99212	OF--Established Patient Low	X
99213	OF--Established Patient Detailed	
99214	OF--Established Patient Moderate	
99215	OF--Established Patient High	
PREVENTIVE VISITS - NEW		
99381	Under 1 Year	
99382	1 - 4 Years	
99383	5 - 11 Years	
99384	12 - 17 Years	
99385	18 - 39 Years	
99386	40 - 64 Years	
99387	65 Years & Up	
PREVENTIVE VISITS - ESTABLISHED		
99391	Under 1 Year	
99392	1 - 4 Years	
99393	5 - 11 Years	
99394	12 - 17 Years	
99395	18 - 39 Years	
99396	40 - 64 Years	
99397	65 Years & Up	
PROCEDURES		
12011	Repair of superficial wounds, face	
29125	Short arm splint	
45378	Colonoscopy--diagnostic	
45380	Colonoscopy--biopsy	
71010	Chest x-ray, frontal	
71020	Chest x-ray, frontal and lateral	
73070	Elbow x-ray, AP and lateral	

PROCEDURES		
73090	Forearm x-ray, AP and lateral	
73100	Wrist x-ray, AP and lateral	
73600	Ankle x-ray, AP and lateral	
93000	Electrocardiogram--ECG	
93015	Treadmill stress test	
LABORATORY		
80061	Lipid panel	
82270	Hemoccult--stool screening	
82465	Cholesterol test	
82947	Glucose--quantitative	
82951	Glucose tolerance test	
83718	HDL cholesterol test	
85007	Manual WBC	
85025	CBC w/diff.	
85651	Erythrocyte sed rate--ESR	
86580	Mantoux test	
87040	Bacterial culture	
87430	Strep screen	
87086	Urine colony count	X
87088	Urine culture	
INJECTIONS		
90465	Immunization administration, pt under 8 yrs	
90471	Immunization administration	
90657	Influenza injection, under 35 months	
90658	Influenza injection, older than 3 years	
90703	Tetanus immunization	
90707	MMR immunization	

PB FAMILY CARE CENTER

REFERRING PHYSICIAN	NPI
AUTHORIZATION #	

NOTES

DIAGNOSIS
599.0 urinary tract infection

PAYMENT AMOUNT
$15 copayment, check #2011

ENCOUNTER FORM

11/3/10 DATE	**10:15am** TIME

Dr. Katherine Yan
PROVIDER

Ellen Barmenstein
PATIENT NAME

BAREL000
CHART #

OFFICE VISITS - SYMPTOMATIC - NEW		
99201	OF--New Patient Minimal	
99202	OF--New Patient Low	
99203	OF--New Patient Detailed	
99204	OF--New Patient Moderate	
99205	OF--New Patient High	
OFFICE VISITS - SYMPTOMATIC - ESTABLISHED		
99211	OF--Established Patient Minimal	X
99212	OF--Established Patient Low	
99213	OF--Established Patient Detailed	
99214	OF--Established Patient Moderate	
99215	OF--Established Patient High	
PREVENTIVE VISITS - NEW		
99381	Under 1 Year	
99382	1 - 4 Years	
99383	5 - 11 Years	
99384	12 - 17 Years	
99385	18 - 39 Years	
99386	40 - 64 Years	
99387	65 Years & Up	
PREVENTIVE VISITS - ESTABLISHED		
99391	Under 1 Year	
99392	1 - 4 Years	
99393	5 - 11 Years	
99394	12 - 17 Years	
99395	18 - 39 Years	
99396	40 - 64 Years	
99397	65 Years & Up	
PROCEDURES		
12011	Repair of superficial wounds, face	
29125	Short arm splint	
45378	Colonoscopy--diagnostic	
45380	Colonoscopy--biopsy	
71010	Chest x-ray, frontal	
71020	Chest x-ray, frontal and lateral	
73070	Elbow x-ray, AP and lateral	

PROCEDURES		
73090	Forearm x-ray, AP and lateral	
73100	Wrist x-ray, AP and lateral	
73600	Ankle x-ray, AP and lateral	
93000	Electrocardiogram--ECG	
93015	Treadmill stress test	
LABORATORY		
80061	Lipid panel	
82270	Hemoccult--stool screening	
82465	Cholesterol test	
82947	Glucose--quantitative	
82951	Glucose tolerance test	
83718	HDL cholesterol test	X
85007	Manual WBC	
85025	CBC w/diff.	
85651	Erythrocyte sed rate--ESR	
86580	Mantoux test	
87040	Bacterial culture	
87430	Strep screen	
87086	Urine colony count	
87088	Urine culture	
INJECTIONS		
90465	Immunization administration, pt under 8 yrs	
90471	Immunization administration	
90657	Influenza injection, under 35 months	
90658	Influenza injection, older than 3 years	
90703	Tetanus immunization	
90707	MMR immunization	

PB FAMILY CARE CENTER

REFERRING PHYSICIAN	NPI
AUTHORIZATION #	
DIAGNOSIS 272.0 hypercholesterolemia	
PAYMENT AMOUNT	

NOTES

ENCOUNTER FORM

11/3/10   10:30am
DATE   TIME

Elizabeth Jones
PATIENT NAME

Dr. Katherine Yan
PROVIDER

JONEL000
CHART #

OFFICE VISITS - SYMPTOMATIC - NEW		
99201	OF--New Patient Minimal	
99202	OF--New Patient Low	
99203	OF--New Patient Detailed	
99204	OF--New Patient Moderate	
99205	OF--New Patient High	
OFFICE VISITS - SYMPTOMATIC - ESTABLISHED		
99211	OF--Established Patient Minimal	
99212	OF--Established Patient Low	X
99213	OF--Established Patient Detailed	
99214	OF--Established Patient Moderate	
99215	OF--Established Patient High	
PREVENTIVE VISITS - NEW		
99381	Under 1 Year	
99382	1 - 4 Years	
99383	5 - 11 Years	
99384	12 - 17 Years	
99385	18 - 39 Years	
99386	40 - 64 Years	
99387	65 Years & Up	
PREVENTIVE VISITS - ESTABLISHED		
99391	Under 1 Year	
99392	1 - 4 Years	
99393	5 - 11 Years	
99394	12 - 17 Years	
99395	18 - 39 Years	
99396	40 - 64 Years	
99397	65 Years & Up	
PROCEDURES		
12011	Repair of superficial wounds, face	
29125	Short arm splint	
45378	Colonoscopy--diagnostic	
45380	Colonoscopy--biopsy	
71010	Chest x-ray, frontal	
71020	Chest x-ray, frontal and lateral	
73070	Elbow x-ray, AP and lateral	

PROCEDURES		
73090	Forearm x-ray, AP and lateral	
73100	Wrist x-ray, AP and lateral	
73600	Ankle x-ray, AP and lateral	
93000	Electrocardiogram--ECG	
93015	Treadmill stress test	
LABORATORY		
80061	Lipid panel	
82270	Hemoccult--stool screening	
82465	Cholesterol test	
82947	Glucose--quantitative	
82951	Glucose tolerance test	
83718	HDL cholesterol test	
85007	Manual WBC	
85025	CBC w/diff.	
85651	Erythrocyte sed rate--ESR	
86580	Mantoux test	
87040	Bacterial culture	
87430	Strep screen	
87086	Urine colony count	
87088	Urine culture	
INJECTIONS		
90465	Immunization administration, pt under 8 yrs	
90471	Immunization administration	
90657	Influenza injection, under 35 months	
90658	Influenza injection, older than 3 years	
90703	Tetanus immunization	
90707	MMR immunization	

PB FAMILY CARE CENTER

REFERRING PHYSICIAN	NPI
AUTHORIZATION #	

DIAGNOSIS
461.9 acute sinusitis

PAYMENT AMOUNT
$15 copayment, check #4226

NOTES

ENCOUNTER FORM

11/3/10	2:00pm	Dr. Katherine Yan
DATE	TIME	PROVIDER

James L. Smith	SMIJA000
PATIENT NAME	CHART #

OFFICE VISITS - SYMPTOMATIC - NEW		
99201	OF--New Patient Minimal	
99202	OF--New Patient Low	
99203	OF--New Patient Detailed	
99204	OF--New Patient Moderate	
99205	OF--New Patient High	
OFFICE VISITS - SYMPTOMATIC - ESTABLISHED		
99211	OF--Established Patient Minimal	
99212	OF--Established Patient Low	
99213	OF--Established Patient Detailed	
99214	OF--Established Patient Moderate	X
99215	OF--Established Patient High	
PREVENTIVE VISITS - NEW		
99381	Under 1 Year	
99382	1 - 4 Years	
99383	5 - 11 Years	
99384	12 - 17 Years	
99385	18 - 39 Years	
99386	40 - 64 Years	
99387	65 Years & Up	
PREVENTIVE VISITS - ESTABLISHED		
99391	Under 1 Year	
99392	1 - 4 Years	
99393	5 - 11 Years	
99394	12 - 17 Years	
99395	18 - 39 Years	
99396	40 - 64 Years	
99397	65 Years & Up	
PROCEDURES		
12011	Repair of superficial wounds, face	
29125	Short arm splint	
45378	Colonoscopy--diagnostic	
45380	Colonoscopy--biopsy	
71010	Chest x-ray, frontal	
71020	Chest x-ray, frontal and lateral	
73070	Elbow x-ray, AP and lateral	

PROCEDURES		
73090	Forearm x-ray, AP and lateral	
73100	Wrist x-ray, AP and lateral	
73600	Ankle x-ray, AP and lateral	
93000	Electrocardiogram--ECG	X
93015	Treadmill stress test	X
LABORATORY		
80061	Lipid panel	
82270	Hemoccult--stool screening	
82465	Cholesterol test	
82947	Glucose--quantitative	
82951	Glucose tolerance test	
83718	HDL cholesterol test	
85007	Manual WBC	
85025	CBC w/diff.	
85651	Erythrocyte sed rate--ESR	
86580	Mantoux test	
87040	Bacterial culture	
87430	Strep screen	
87086	Urine colony count	
87088	Urine culture	
INJECTIONS		
90465	Immunization administration, pt under 8 yrs	
90471	Immunization administration	
90657	Influenza injection, under 35 months	
90658	Influenza injection, older than 3 years	
90703	Tetanus immunization	
90707	MMR immunization	

PB FAMILY CARE CENTER		NOTES
REFERRING PHYSICIAN	NPI	
AUTHORIZATION #		
DIAGNOSIS		
786.50 chest pain		
PAYMENT AMOUNT		

PATIENT INFORMATION FORM

THIS SECTION REFERS TO PATIENT ONLY

Name: Joe Abate	Sex: M	Marital Status: ☐S ☒M ☐D ☐W	Birth Date: 10/1/67

Address: 86 Western Drive	SS#: 403-53-3491

City: Stephenson	State: OH	Zip: 60089	Employer: Stephenson Wire Works (full-time)

Home Phone: 614-931-3317	Employer's Address:

Work Phone: 614-525-0215	City:	State:	Zip:

Spouse's Name:	Spouse's Employer:

Emergency Contact:	Relationship:	Phone #:

FILL IN IF PATIENT IS A MINOR

Parent/Guardian's Name:	Sex:	Marital Status: ☐S ☐M ☐D ☐W	Birth Date:

Phone:	SS#:

Address:	Employer:

City:	State:	Zip:	Employer's Address:

Student Status:	City:	State:	Zip:

INSURANCE INFORMATION

Primary Insurance Company: Physician's Choice	Secondary Insurance Company:

Subscriber's Name: (same)	Birth Date: 10/1/67	Subscriber's Name:	Birth Date:

Plan:	SS#: 403-53-3491	Plan:

Policy #: 321728	Group #: E4362	Policy #:	Group #:

Copayment: $15	Deductible:	Price Code: A

OTHER INFORMATION

Reason for visit: Preventive exam	Allergy to Medication (list):

Name of referring physician:	If auto accident, list date and state in which it occurred:

I authorize treatment and agree to pay all fees and charges for the person named above. I agree to pay all charges shown by statements, promptly upon their presentation, unless credit arrangements are agreed upon in writing.

I authorize payment directly to FAMILY CARE CENTER of insurance benefits otherwise payable to me. I hereby authorize the release of any medical information necessary in order to process a claim for payment in my behalf.

Joe Abate	11/3/10
(Patient's Signature/Parent or Guardian's Signature)	(Date)

I plan to make payment of my medical expenses as follows (check one or more):

__X__ Insurance (as above)   __X__ Cash/Check/Credit/Debit Card   _____ Medicare   _____ Medicaid   _____ Workers'

ENCOUNTER FORM

11/3/10 2:30pm	Dr. Katherine Yan
DATE TIME	PROVIDER
Joe Abate	ABAJO000
PATIENT NAME	CHART #

OFFICE VISITS - SYMPTOMATIC - NEW		
99201	OF--New Patient Minimal	
99202	OF--New Patient Low	
99203	OF--New Patient Detailed	
99204	OF--New Patient Moderate	
99205	OF--New Patient High	

OFFICE VISITS - SYMPTOMATIC - ESTABLISHED		
99211	OF--Established Patient Minimal	
99212	OF--Established Patient Low	
99213	OF--Established Patient Detailed	
99214	OF--Established Patient Moderate	
99215	OF--Established Patient High	

PREVENTIVE VISITS - NEW		
99381	Under 1 Year	
99382	1 - 4 Years	
99383	5 - 11 Years	
99384	12 - 17 Years	
99385	18 - 39 Years	
99386	40 - 64 Years	X
99387	65 Years & Up	

PREVENTIVE VISITS - ESTABLISHED		
99391	Under 1 Year	
99392	1 - 4 Years	
99393	5 - 11 Years	
99394	12 - 17 Years	
99395	18 - 39 Years	
99396	40 - 64 Years	
99397	65 Years & Up	

PROCEDURES		
12011	Repair of superficial wounds, face	
29125	Short arm splint	
45378	Colonoscopy--diagnostic	
45380	Colonoscopy--biopsy	
71010	Chest x-ray, frontal	
71020	Chest x-ray, frontal and lateral	
73070	Elbow x-ray, AP and lateral	

PROCEDURES		
73090	Forearm x-ray, AP and lateral	
73100	Wrist x-ray, AP and lateral	
73600	Ankle x-ray, AP and lateral	
93000	Electrocardiogram--ECG	
93015	Treadmill stress test	

LABORATORY		
80061	Lipid panel	
82270	Hemoccult--stool screening	
82465	Cholesterol test	
82947	Glucose--quantitative	
82951	Glucose tolerance test	
83718	HDL cholesterol test	
85007	Manual WBC	
85025	CBC w/diff.	
85651	Erythrocyte sed rate--ESR	
86580	Mantoux test	
87040	Bacterial culture	
87430	Strep screen	
87086	Urine colony count	
87088	Urine culture	

INJECTIONS		
90465	Immunization administration, pt under 8 yrs	
90471	Immunization administration	
90657	Influenza injection, under 35 months	
90658	Influenza injection, older than 3 years	
90703	Tetanus immunization	
90707	MMR immunization	

PB FAMILY CARE CENTER		NOTES
REFERRING PHYSICIAN	NPI	
AUTHORIZATION #		
DIAGNOSIS		
v70.0 adult physical examination		
PAYMENT AMOUNT		
$15 copayment, check #124		

ENCOUNTER FORM

11/3/10	3:00pm
DATE	TIME

Dr. Katherine Yan
PROVIDER

Sarabeth Smith
PATIENT NAME

SMISA000
CHART #

OFFICE VISITS - SYMPTOMATIC - NEW		
99201	OF--New Patient Minimal	
99202	OF--New Patient Low	
99203	OF--New Patient Detailed	
99204	OF--New Patient Moderate	
99205	OF--New Patient High	
OFFICE VISITS - SYMPTOMATIC - ESTABLISHED		
99211	OF--Established Patient Minimal	
99212	OF--Established Patient Low	
99213	OF--Established Patient Detailed	
99214	OF--Established Patient Moderate	
99215	OF--Established Patient High	
PREVENTIVE VISITS - NEW		
99381	Under 1 Year	
99382	1 - 4 Years	
99383	5 - 11 Years	
99384	12 - 17 Years	
99385	18 - 39 Years	
99386	40 - 64 Years	
99387	65 Years & Up	
PREVENTIVE VISITS - ESTABLISHED		
99391	Under 1 Year	
99392	1 - 4 Years	
99393	5 - 11 Years	
99394	12 - 17 Years	
99395	18 - 39 Years	X
99396	40 - 64 Years	
99397	65 Years & Up	
PROCEDURES		
12011	Repair of superficial wounds, face	
29125	Short arm splint	
45378	Colonoscopy--diagnostic	
45380	Colonoscopy--biopsy	
71010	Chest x-ray, frontal	
71020	Chest x-ray, frontal and lateral	
73070	Elbow x-ray, AP and lateral	

PROCEDURES		
73090	Forearm x-ray, AP and lateral	
73100	Wrist x-ray, AP and lateral	
73600	Ankle x-ray, AP and lateral	
93000	Electrocardiogram--ECG	
93015	Treadmill stress test	
LABORATORY		
80061	Lipid panel	
82270	Hemoccult--stool screening	
82465	Cholesterol test	
82947	Glucose--quantitative	
82951	Glucose tolerance test	
83718	HDL cholesterol test	
85007	Manual WBC	
85025	CBC w/diff.	
85651	Erythrocyte sed rate--ESR	
86580	Mantoux test	
87040	Bacterial culture	
87430	Strep screen	
87086	Urine colony count	
87088	Urine culture	
INJECTIONS		
90465	Immunization administration, pt under 8 yrs	
90471	Immunization administration	
90657	Influenza injection, under 35 months	
90658	Influenza injection, older than 3 years	
90703	Tetanus immunization	
90707	MMR immunization	

PB FAMILY CARE CENTER		NOTES
REFERRING PHYSICIAN	NPI	
AUTHORIZATION #		
DIAGNOSIS		
v70.0 adult physical examination		
PAYMENT AMOUNT		

MARION JOHNSON   No. 1234
3511 WEST STREET
STEPHENSON OH 60089   Date Oct. 29, 2010

PAYABLE TO   Family Care Center $61.20

Sixty-one and 20/100 ——————————————————————— dollars

Stephenson Bank
Stephenson, OH 60089   _____
                                             Marion Johnson

021203347   0379 399 34   1234

U.S. Life
2788 Broadway
New York, NY 10021

PROVIDER REMITTANCE
THIS IS NOT A BILL
A PAYMENT SUMMARY AND AN EXPLANATION OF
CODES ARE AT THE END OF THIS STATEMENT

FAMILY CARE CENTER
285 STEPHENSON BLVD.
STEPHENSON, OH 60089

Date Prepared:	11/3/10
EFT Number:	36805
Amount:	$ 138.00

PROVIDER: KATHERINE YAN, M.D.

PATIENT: SAMPSON, ETHAN

PROC CODE	Date of Service From–Thru	Qty	Amount Charged	Allowed Amount	Copay/ Deduct	Patient Balance	Adjustment	Amt Paid Provider
99214	11/01/10 - 11/01/10	1	85.00	76.50	15.00	0.00	-8.50	61.50
73090	11/01/10 - 11/01/10	1	85.00	76.50	0.00	0.00	-8.50	76.50
	TOTALS		170.00	153.00	15.00	0.00	-17.00	138.00

PAYMENT SUMMARY

TOTAL AMOUNT PAID	138.00
PRIOR CREDIT BALANCE	0.00
CURRENT CREDIT DEFERRED	0.00
PRIOR CREDIT APPLIED	0.00
NEW CREDIT BALANCE	0.00
NET DISBURSED	138.00

TOTAL ALL CLAIMS

AMOUNT CHARGED	170.00
AMOUNT ALLOWED	153.00
DEDUCTIBLE	0.00
COPAY	15.00
OTHER REDUCTION	0.00
AMOUNT APPROVED	138.00

STATUS CODES:
A - APPROVED   AJ - ADJUSTMENT   IP - IN PROCESS   R - REJECTED   V - VOID

Physician's Choice Services
9800 Blue Rock Turnpike
Clarksville OH 60817

PROVIDER REMITTANCE

THIS IS NOT A BILL
A PAYMENT SUMMARY AND AN EXPLANATION OF
CODES ARE AT THE END OF THIS STATEMENT

FAMILY CARE CENTER
285 STEPHENSON BLVD.
STEPHENSON, OH 60089

Date Prepared:	11/3/10
EFT Number:	657104
Amount:	$ 343.50

PROVIDER: KATHERINE YAN, M.D.

PATIENT: ANDREWS, DARLA

PROC CODE	Date of Service From–Thru	Qty	Amount Charged	Allowed Amount	Copay/ Deduct	Patient Balance	Adjustment	Amt Paid Provider
99203	11/01/10 - 11/01/10	1	100.00	90.00	15.00	0.00	-10.00	75.00
71010	11/01/10 - 11/01/10	1	80.00	72.00	0.00	0.00	-8.00	72.00
93000	11/01/10 - 11/01/10	1	70.00	63.00	0.00	0.00	-7.00	63.00
	TOTALS		250.00	225.00	15.00	0.00	-25.00	210.00

PATIENT: ANDREWS, WILLIAM

PROC CODE	Date of Service From–Thru	Qty	Amount Charged	Allowed Amount	Copay/ Deduct	Patient Balance	Adjustment	Amt Paid Provider
99385	11/01/10 - 11/01/10	1	165.00	148.50	15.00	0.00	-16.50	133.50
	TOTALS		165.00	148.50	15.00	0.00	-16.50	133.50

PAYMENT SUMMARY		TOTAL ALL CLAIMS	
TOTAL AMOUNT PAID	343.50	AMOUNT CHARGED	415.00
PRIOR CREDIT BALANCE	0.00	AMOUNT ALLOWED	373.50
CURRENT CREDIT DEFERRED	0.00	DEDUCTIBLE	0.00
PRIOR CREDIT APPLIED	0.00	COPAY	30.00
NEW CREDIT BALANCE	0.00	OTHER REDUCTION	0.00
NET DISBURSED	343.50	AMOUNT APPROVED	343.50

STATUS CODES:
A - APPROVED   AJ - ADJUSTMENT   IP - IN PROCESS   R - REJECTED   V - VOID

ENCOUNTER FORM

11/4/10	9:00am	Dr. Katherine Yan
DATE	TIME	PROVIDER

Maritza Ramos	RAMMA000
PATIENT NAME	CHART #

OFFICE VISITS - SYMPTOMATIC - NEW		
99201	OF--New Patient Minimal	
99202	OF--New Patient Low	
99203	OF--New Patient Detailed	
99204	OF--New Patient Moderate	
99205	OF--New Patient High	
OFFICE VISITS - SYMPTOMATIC - ESTABLISHED		
99211	OF--Established Patient Minimal	X
99212	OF--Established Patient Low	
99213	OF--Established Patient Detailed	
99214	OF--Established Patient Moderate	
99215	OF--Established Patient High	
PREVENTIVE VISITS - NEW		
99381	Under 1 Year	
99382	1 - 4 Years	
99383	5 - 11 Years	
99384	12 - 17 Years	
99385	18 - 39 Years	
99386	40 - 64 Years	
99387	65 Years & Up	
PREVENTIVE VISITS - ESTABLISHED		
99391	Under 1 Year	
99392	1 - 4 Years	
99393	5 - 11 Years	
99394	12 - 17 Years	
99395	18 - 39 Years	
99396	40 - 64 Years	
99397	65 Years & Up	
PROCEDURES		
12011	Repair of superficial wounds, face	
29125	Short arm splint	
45378	Colonoscopy--diagnostic	
45380	Colonoscopy--biopsy	
71010	Chest x-ray, frontal	
71020	Chest x-ray, frontal and lateral	
73070	Elbow x-ray, AP and lateral	

PROCEDURES		
73090	Forearm x-ray, AP and lateral	
73100	Wrist x-ray, AP and lateral	
73600	Ankle x-ray, AP and lateral	
93000	Electrocardiogram--ECG	
93015	Treadmill stress test	
LABORATORY		
80061	Lipid panel	
82270	Hemoccult--stool screening	
82465	Cholesterol test	
82947	Glucose--quantitative	
82951	Glucose tolerance test	
83718	HDL cholesterol test	
85007	Manual WBC	X
85025	CBC w/diff.	
85651	Erythrocyte sed rate--ESR	
86580	Mantoux test	
87040	Bacterial culture	
87430	Strep screen	
87086	Urine colony count	
87088	Urine culture	
INJECTIONS		
90465	Immunization administration, pt under 8 yrs	
90471	Immunization administration	
90657	Influenza injection, under 35 months	
90658	Influenza injection, older than 3 years	
90703	Tetanus immunization	
90707	MMR immunization	

PB FAMILY CARE CENTER

REFERRING PHYSICIAN	NPI

NOTES

AUTHORIZATION #

DIAGNOSIS
487.1 influenza

PAYMENT AMOUNT
$15 copayment, check #1047

ENCOUNTER FORM

11/4/10	9:30am	Dr. Katherine Yan
DATE	TIME	PROVIDER

Sarina Bell	BELSA000
PATIENT NAME	CHART #

OFFICE VISITS - SYMPTOMATIC - NEW		
99201	OF--New Patient Minimal	
99202	OF--New Patient Low	
99203	OF--New Patient Detailed	
99204	OF--New Patient Moderate	
99205	OF--New Patient High	
OFFICE VISITS - SYMPTOMATIC - ESTABLISHED		
99211	OF--Established Patient Minimal	
99212	OF--Established Patient Low	X
99213	OF--Established Patient Detailed	
99214	OF--Established Patient Moderate	
99215	OF--Established Patient High	
PREVENTIVE VISITS - NEW		
99381	Under 1 Year	
99382	1 - 4 Years	
99383	5 - 11 Years	
99384	12 - 17 Years	
99385	18 - 39 Years	
99386	40 - 64 Years	
99387	65 Years & Up	
PREVENTIVE VISITS - ESTABLISHED		
99391	Under 1 Year	
99392	1 - 4 Years	
99393	5 - 11 Years	
99394	12 - 17 Years	
99395	18 - 39 Years	
99396	40 - 64 Years	
99397	65 Years & Up	
PROCEDURES		
12011	Repair of superficial wounds, face	
29125	Short arm splint	
45378	Colonoscopy--diagnostic	
45380	Colonoscopy--biopsy	
71010	Chest x-ray, frontal	
71020	Chest x-ray, frontal and lateral	
73070	Elbow x-ray, AP and lateral	

PROCEDURES		
73090	Forearm x-ray, AP and lateral	
73100	Wrist x-ray, AP and lateral	
73600	Ankle x-ray, AP and lateral	
93000	Electrocardiogram--ECG	
93015	Treadmill stress test	
LABORATORY		
80061	Lipid panel	
82270	Hemoccult--stool screening	
82465	Cholesterol test	
82947	Glucose--quantitative	
82951	Glucose tolerance test	
83718	HDL cholesterol test	
85007	Manual WBC	
85025	CBC w/diff.	
85651	Erythrocyte sed rate--ESR	
86580	Mantoux test	
87040	Bacterial culture	
87430	Strep screen	
87086	Urine colony count	
87088	Urine culture	
INJECTIONS		
90465	Immunization administration, pt under 8 yrs	
90471	Immunization administration	
90657	Influenza injection, under 35 months	
90658	Influenza injection, older than 3 years	
90703	Tetanus immunization	
90707	MMR immunization	

PB FAMILY CARE CENTER

REFERRING PHYSICIAN	NPI	NOTES
AUTHORIZATION #		
DIAGNOSIS 461.9 acute sinusitis		
PAYMENT AMOUNT $15 copayment, check #3126		

ENCOUNTER FORM

11/4/10	**10:00am**
DATE	TIME

Dr. Katherine Yan
PROVIDER

Jo Wong
PATIENT NAME

WONJO000
CHART #

OFFICE VISITS - SYMPTOMATIC - NEW		
99201	OF--New Patient Minimal	
99202	OF--New Patient Low	
99203	OF--New Patient Detailed	
99204	OF--New Patient Moderate	
99205	OF--New Patient High	
OFFICE VISITS - SYMPTOMATIC - ESTABLISHED		
99211	OF--Established Patient Minimal	X
99212	OF--Established Patient Low	
99213	OF--Established Patient Detailed	
99214	OF--Established Patient Moderate	
99215	OF--Established Patient High	
PREVENTIVE VISITS - NEW		
99381	Under 1 Year	
99382	1 - 4 Years	
99383	5 - 11 Years	
99384	12 - 17 Years	
99385	18 - 39 Years	
99386	40 - 64 Years	
99387	65 Years & Up	
PREVENTIVE VISITS - ESTABLISHED		
99391	Under 1 Year	
99392	1 - 4 Years	
99393	5 - 11 Years	
99394	12 - 17 Years	
99395	18 - 39 Years	
99396	40 - 64 Years	
99397	65 Years & Up	
PROCEDURES		
12011	Repair of superficial wounds, face	
29125	Short arm splint	
45378	Colonoscopy--diagnostic	
45380	Colonoscopy--biopsy	
71010	Chest x-ray, frontal	
71020	Chest x-ray, frontal and lateral	
73070	Elbow x-ray, AP and lateral	

PROCEDURES		
73090	Forearm x-ray, AP and lateral	
73100	Wrist x-ray, AP and lateral	
73600	Ankle x-ray, AP and lateral	
93000	Electrocardiogram--ECG	
93015	Treadmill stress test	
LABORATORY		
80061	Lipid panel	
82270	Hemoccult--stool screening	
82465	Cholesterol test	
82947	Glucose--quantitative	
82951	Glucose tolerance test	
83718	HDL cholesterol test	
85007	Manual WBC	
85025	CBC w/diff.	
85651	Erythrocyte sed rate--ESR	
86580	Mantoux test	
87040	Bacterial culture	
87430	Strep screen	
87086	Urine colony count	
87088	Urine culture	
INJECTIONS		
90465	Immunization administration, pt under 8 yrs	
90471	Immunization administration	
90657	Influenza injection, under 35 months	
90658	Influenza injection, older than 3 years	
90703	Tetanus immunization	
90707	MMR immunization	

PB FAMILY CARE CENTER		NOTES
REFERRING PHYSICIAN	NPI	
AUTHORIZATION #		
DIAGNOSIS		
v65.5 normal state		
PAYMENT AMOUNT		

BLUE CROSS BLUE SHIELD
340 Preston Boulevard
Columbus, OH 60220

PROVIDER REMITTANCE
THIS IS NOT A BILL
A PAYMENT SUMMARY AND AN EXPLANATION OF
CODES ARE AT THE END OF THIS STATEMENT

FAMILY CARE CENTER
285 STEPHENSON BLVD.
STEPHENSON, OH 60089

Date Prepared:	11/4/10
EFT Number:	36097869
Amount:	$ 364.80

PROVIDER: KATHERINE YAN, M.D.

PATIENT: BLACK, JO

PROC CODE	Date of Service From–Thru	Qty	Amount Charged	Allowed Amount	Copay/ Deduct	Patient Balance	Adjustment	Amt Paid Provider
99203	11/01/10 - 11/01/10	1	100.00	100.00	0.00	20.00	0.00	80.00
93000	11/01/10 - 11/01/10	1	70.00	70.00	0.00	14.00	0.00	56.00
	TOTALS		170.00	170.00	0.00	34.00	0.00	136.00

PATIENT: FELDMAN, STANLEY

PROC CODE	Date of Service From–Thru	Qty	Amount Charged	Allowed Amount	Copay/ Deduct	Patient Balance	Adjustment	Amt Paid Provider
99211	11/01/10 - 11/01/10	1	30.00	30.00	0.00	6.00	0.00	24.00
80061	11/01/10 - 11/01/10	1	70.00	70.00	0.00	14.00	0.00	56.00
	TOTALS		100.00	100.00	0.00	20.00	0.00	80.00

PATIENT: JOHNSON, MARION

PROC CODE	Date of Service From–Thru	Qty	Amount Charged	Allowed Amount	Copay/ Deduct	Patient Balance	Adjustment	Amt Paid Provider
99212	10/29/10 - 10/29/10	1	44.00	44.00	0.00	8.80	0.00	35.20
71010	10/29/10 - 10/29/10	1	80.00	80.00	0.00	16.00	0.00	64.00
87430	10/29/10 - 10/29/10	1	32.00	32.00	0.00	6.40	0.00	25.60
	TOTALS		156.00	156.00	0.00	31.20	0.00	124.80

PATIENT: LOMOS, CEDERA

PROC CODE	Date of Service From–Thru	Qty	Amount Charged	Allowed Amount	Copay/ Deduct	Patient Balance	Adjustment	Amt Paid Provider
99211	11/01/10 - 11/01/10	1	30.00	30.00	0.00	6.00	0.00	24.00
	TOTALS		30.00	30.00	0.00	6.00	0.00	24.00

PAYMENT SUMMARY

TOTAL AMOUNT PAID	364.80
PRIOR CREDIT BALANCE	0.00
CURRENT CREDIT DEFERRED	0.00
PRIOR CREDIT APPLIED	0.00
NEW CREDIT BALANCE	0.00
NET DISBURSED	364.80

TOTAL ALL CLAIMS

AMOUNT CHARGED	456.00
AMOUNT ALLOWED	456.00
DEDUCTIBLE	0.00
COPAY	0.00
OTHER REDUCTION	0.00
AMOUNT APPROVED	364.80

STATUS CODES:
A - APPROVED   AJ - ADJUSTMENT   IP - IN PROCESS   R - REJECTED   V - VOID

JAMES L. SMITH
17 BLACKS LANE
STEPHENSON OH 60089

No. 6789

Date Oct. 29, 2010

PAYABLE TO   Family Care Center

$17.60

Seventeen and 60/100 ——————————————————————— dollars

Stephenson Bank
Stephenson, OH 60089

James L. Smith

021203347   0379 400 12   6789

PATIENT INFORMATION FORM

THIS SECTION REFERS TO PATIENT ONLY

Name: Uzwahl, Surendra	Sex: F Marital Status: ☐S ☐M ☒D ☐W Birth Date: 7/8/68

Address: 15 Main Street	SS#: 393-59-4392

City: Stephenson	State: OH	Zip: 60089	Employer: J.C. Penney (full-time)

Home Phone: 614-931-3715	Employer's Address:

Work Phone: 614-344-3118	City: State: Zip:

Spouse's Name:	Spouse's Employer:

Emergency Contact:	Relationship: Phone #:

FILL IN IF PATIENT IS A MINOR

Parent/Guardian's Name:	Sex: Marital Status: ☐S ☐M ☐D ☐W Birth Date:
Phone:	SS#:
Address:	Employer:
City: State: Zip:	Employer's Address:
Student Status:	City: State: Zip:

INSURANCE INFORMATION

Primary Insurance Company: Blue Cross/Blue Shield	Secondary Insurance Company:
Subscriber's Name: (same) Birth Date: 7/8/68	Subscriber's Name: Birth Date:
Plan: SS#: 393-59-4392	Plan:
Policy #: 393594392 Group #: 36	Policy #: Group #:

Copayment:	Deductible: $500	Price Code: A

OTHER INFORMATION

Reason for visit: Ankle hurt in fall	Allergy to Medication (list):
Name of referring physician:	If auto accident, list date and state in which it occurred:

I authorize treatment and agree to pay all fees and charges for the person named above. I agree to pay all charges shown by statements, promptly upon their presentation, unless credit arrangements are agreed upon in writing.

I authorize payment directly to FAMILY CARE CENTER of insurance benefits otherwise payable to me. I hereby authorize the release of any medical information necessary in order to process a claim for payment in my behalf.

Surendra Uzwahl	11/5/10
(Patient's Signature/Parent or Guardian's Signature)	(Date)

I plan to make payment of my medical expenses as follows (check one or more):

<u>X</u> Insurance (as above)   <u>X</u> Cash/Check/Credit/Debit Card   _____ Medicare   _____ Medicaid   _____ Workers' Comp.

ENCOUNTER FORM

11/5/10	9:00am	Dr. Katherine Yan
DATE	TIME	PROVIDER

Surendra Uzwahl	UZWSU000
PATIENT NAME	CHART #

OFFICE VISITS - SYMPTOMATIC - NEW		
99201	OF--New Patient Minimal	
99202	OF--New Patient Low	X
99203	OF--New Patient Detailed	
99204	OF--New Patient Moderate	
99205	OF--New Patient High	
OFFICE VISITS - SYMPTOMATIC - ESTABLISHED		
99211	OF--Established Patient Minimal	
99212	OF--Established Patient Low	
99213	OF--Established Patient Detailed	
99214	OF--Established Patient Moderate	
99215	OF--Established Patient High	
PREVENTIVE VISITS - NEW		
99381	Under 1 Year	
99382	1 - 4 Years	
99383	5 - 11 Years	
99384	12 - 17 Years	
99385	18 - 39 Years	
99386	40 - 64 Years	
99387	65 Years & Up	
PREVENTIVE VISITS - ESTABLISHED		
99391	Under 1 Year	
99392	1 - 4 Years	
99393	5 - 11 Years	
99394	12 - 17 Years	
99395	18 - 39 Years	
99396	40 - 64 Years	
99397	65 Years & Up	
PROCEDURES		
12011	Repair of superficial wounds, face	
29125	Short arm splint	
45378	Colonoscopy--diagnostic	
45380	Colonoscopy--biopsy	
71010	Chest x-ray, frontal	
71020	Chest x-ray, frontal and lateral	
73070	Elbow x-ray, AP and lateral	

PROCEDURES		
73090	Forearm x-ray, AP and lateral	
73100	Wrist x-ray, AP and lateral	
73600	Ankle x-ray, AP and lateral	X
93000	Electrocardiogram--ECG	
93015	Treadmill stress test	
LABORATORY		
80061	Lipid panel	
82270	Hemoccult--stool screening	
82465	Cholesterol test	
82947	Glucose--quantitative	
82951	Glucose tolerance test	
83718	HDL cholesterol test	
85007	Manual WBC	
85025	CBC w/diff.	
85651	Erythrocyte sed rate--ESR	
86580	Mantoux test	
87040	Bacterial culture	
87430	Strep screen	
87086	Urine colony count	
87088	Urine culture	
INJECTIONS		
90465	Immunization administration, pt under 8 yrs	
90471	Immunization administration	
90657	Influenza injection, under 35 months	
90658	Influenza injection, older than 3 years	
90703	Tetanus immunization	
90707	MMR immunization	

PB FAMILY CARE CENTER		NOTES
REFERRING PHYSICIAN	NPI	
AUTHORIZATION #		
DIAGNOSIS		
848.9 sprain		
PAYMENT AMOUNT		

ENCOUNTER FORM

11/5/10	**9:30am**
DATE	TIME

Dr. Katherine Yan
PROVIDER

Jonathan Bell
PATIENT NAME

BELJO000
CHART #

OFFICE VISITS - SYMPTOMATIC - NEW		
99201	OF--New Patient Minimal	
99202	OF--New Patient Low	
99203	OF--New Patient Detailed	
99204	OF--New Patient Moderate	
99205	OF--New Patient High	

OFFICE VISITS - SYMPTOMATIC - ESTABLISHED		
99211	OF--Established Patient Minimal	
99212	OF--Established Patient Low	X
99213	OF--Established Patient Detailed	
99214	OF--Established Patient Moderate	
99215	OF--Established Patient High	

PREVENTIVE VISITS - NEW		
99381	Under 1 Year	
99382	1 - 4 Years	
99383	5 - 11 Years	
99384	12 - 17 Years	
99385	18 - 39 Years	
99386	40 - 64 Years	
99387	65 Years & Up	

PREVENTIVE VISITS - ESTABLISHED		
99391	Under 1 Year	
99392	1 - 4 Years	
99393	5 - 11 Years	
99394	12 - 17 Years	
99395	18 - 39 Years	
99396	40 - 64 Years	
99397	65 Years & Up	

PROCEDURES		
12011	Repair of superficial wounds, face	
29125	Short arm splint	
45378	Colonoscopy--diagnostic	
45380	Colonoscopy--biopsy	
71010	Chest x-ray, frontal	
71020	Chest x-ray, frontal and lateral	
73070	Elbow x-ray, AP and lateral	

PROCEDURES		
73090	Forearm x-ray, AP and lateral	
73100	Wrist x-ray, AP and lateral	
73600	Ankle x-ray, AP and lateral	
93000	Electrocardiogram--ECG	
93015	Treadmill stress test	

LABORATORY		
80061	Lipid panel	
82270	Hemoccult--stool screening	
82465	Cholesterol test	
82947	Glucose--quantitative	
82951	Glucose tolerance test	
83718	HDL cholesterol test	
85007	Manual WBC	
85025	CBC w/diff.	
85651	Erythrocyte sed rate--ESR	
86580	Mantoux test	
87040	Bacterial culture	
87430	Strep screen	
87086	Urine colony count	
87088	Urine culture	

INJECTIONS		
90465	Immunization administration, pt under 8 yrs	
90471	Immunization administration	
90657	Influenza injection, under 35 months	
90658	Influenza injection, older than 3 years	
90703	Tetanus immunization	
90707	MMR immunization	

PB FAMILY CARE CENTER		NOTES
REFERRING PHYSICIAN	NPI	
AUTHORIZATION #		
DIAGNOSIS **487.1 influenza**		
PAYMENT AMOUNT **$15 copayment, check #6130**		

U.S. Life
2788 Broadway
New York, NY 10021

PROVIDER REMITTANCE
THIS IS NOT A BILL
A PAYMENT SUMMARY AND AN EXPLANATION OF
CODES ARE AT THE END OF THIS STATEMENT

FAMILY CARE CENTER
285 STEPHENSON BLVD.
STEPHENSON, OH 60089

Date Prepared: 11/5/10
EFT Number: 38529
Amount: $ 225.60

PROVIDER: KATHERINE YAN, M.D.

PATIENT: WU, SAM

PROC CODE	Date of Service From–Thru	Qty	Amount Charged	Allowed Amount	Copay/ Deduct	Patient Balance	Adjustment	Amt Paid Provider
99202	11/03/10 - 11/03/10	1	70.00	63.00	15.00	0.00	-7.00	48.00
73070	11/03/10 - 11/03/10	1	85.00	76.50	0.00	0.00	-8.50	76.50
73090	11/03/10 - 11/03/10	1	85.00	76.50	0.00	0.00	-8.50	76.50
	TOTALS		240.00	216.00	15.00	0.00	-24.00	201.00

PATIENT: JONES, ELIZABETH

PROC CODE	Date of Service From–Thru	Qty	Amount Charged	Allowed Amount	Copay/ Deduct	Patient Balance	Adjustment	Amt Paid Provider
99212	11/03/10 - 11/03/10	1	44.00	39.60	15.00	0.00	-4.40	24.60
	TOTALS		44.00	39.60	15.00	0.00	-4.40	24.60

PAYMENT SUMMARY

TOTAL AMOUNT PAID	225.60
PRIOR CREDIT BALANCE	0.00
CURRENT CREDIT DEFERRED	0.00
PRIOR CREDIT APPLIED	0.00
NEW CREDIT BALANCE	0.00
NET DISBURSED	225.60

TOTAL ALL CLAIMS

AMOUNT CHARGED	284.00
AMOUNT ALLOWED	255.60
DEDUCTIBLE	0.00
COPAY	30.00
OTHER REDUCTION	0.00
AMOUNT APPROVED	225.60

STATUS CODES:
A - APPROVED   AJ - ADJUSTMENT   IP - IN PROCESS   R - REJECTED   V - VOID

Physician's Choice Services
9800 Blue Rock Turnpike
Clarksville OH 60817

PROVIDER REMITTANCE
THIS IS NOT A BILL
A PAYMENT SUMMARY AND AN EXPLANATION OF
CODES ARE AT THE END OF THIS STATEMENT

FAMILY CARE CENTER
285 STEPHENSON BLVD.
STEPHENSON, OH 60089

Date Prepared:	11/5/10
EFT Number:	659620
Amount:	$ 12.00

PROVIDER: KATHERINE YAN, M.D.

PATIENT: GARDINER, JOHN

PROC CODE	Date of Service From–Thru	Qty	Amount Charged	Allowed Amount	Copay/ Deduct	Patient Balance	Adjustment	Amt Paid Provider
99211	11/03/10 - 11/03/10	1	30.00	27.00	15.00	0.00	-3.00	12.00
	TOTALS		30.00	27.00	15.00	0.00	-3.00	12.00

PAYMENT SUMMARY

TOTAL AMOUNT PAID	12.00
PRIOR CREDIT BALANCE	0.00
CURRENT CREDIT DEFERRED	0.00
PRIOR CREDIT APPLIED	0.00
NEW CREDIT BALANCE	0.00
NET DISBURSED	12.00

TOTAL ALL CLAIMS

AMOUNT CHARGED	30.00
AMOUNT ALLOWED	27.00
DEDUCTIBLE	0.00
COPAY	15.00
OTHER REDUCTION	0.00
AMOUNT APPROVED	12.00

STATUS CODES:
A - APPROVED   AJ - ADJUSTMENT   IP - IN PROCESS   R - REJECTED   V - VOID

Glossary

A

Accounting cycle The flow of financial transactions in a business.

Accounts receivable (AR) Monies that are coming into the business.

Adjustment A positive or negative amount entered to correct a patient's account balance.

Aging The classification of accounts receivable by the length of time an account is past due.

B

Backup data A copy of data files at a specific point in time that can be used to restore data to the system.

Billing/Payment Status report A report that lists the status of all transactions having a responsible insurance carrier, showing who has paid and who has not been billed.

C

Capitated plan Type of insurance that pays providers a fixed amount for each patient regardless of the actual medical services received.

Case A grouping of procedures or transactions generally organized by the type of treatment or insurance carrier.

Case billing code A code used to group or organize patients for billing purposes, such as M for Medicare or C for cash patient.

Cash flow Movement of money from patients into a practice and to suppliers and staff out of a practice. Refers to actual cash as opposed to receivables and payables.

Cash payments journal Record of all cash payments, frequently in the form of a checkbook register.

Cash receipts journal Record of all cash received by a business.

CHAMPVA A government health insurance plan for disabled veterans.

Charge The amount (or cost) of a procedure performed by a provider.

Chart number A unique number that identifies each patient, used on all documents that pertain to that patient in Medisoft.

Claim status The current disposition of a medical claim.

Clearinghouse A service bureau that collects electronic media claims from many different medical practices, formats them as necessary, and forwards them to the appropriate insurance carriers.

CMS-1500 A paper insurance form accepted by government insurance plans in some states and by most private insurers (formerly HCFA-1500).

Consumer-driven health plan (CDHP) A plan in which a high-deductible/low-premium insurance plan is combined with a pretax savings account to cover out-of-pocket medical expenses.

Copayment Standard fee set up by an insurance carrier that the patient pays to the provider at the time the medical services are rendered.

CPT-4 Listing of codes for medical services or procedures.

Cycle billing A patient billing system in which patients are divided into groups and statement printing and mailing is staggered throughout the month.

D

Data file A subset of data that is part of a larger database.

Database A collection of information (data) arranged logically so that it can be stored and retrieved.

Day sheet Daily record of activities, patients treated, fees charged, and payments received.

Default An entry automatically displayed in an input field, which can be overwritten.

Diagnosis The physician's determination of what is wrong with the patient, based on an examination.

E

EDI receiver An insurance company or clearinghouse set up to electronically receive and process insurance claims submitted by the medical practice.

Encounter form Record of one patient's visit showing procedures performed, charges, and diagnosis. In a manual system, this document may also be referred to as a fee slip, routing slip, or superbill.

EPSDT (Early and Periodic Screening, Diagnosis, and Treatment) Well-baby program sponsored by Medicaid.

Established patient A patient who has received medical care from a physician in the practice in the last three years.

G

General ledger Record of all the accounts of a business.

Global coverage period Specified period of time during which all transactions for a case with a surgical procedure charge default to a zero charge because the initial charge automatically includes the follow-up work.

Guarantor The person or third party responsible for payment of a patient's medical bills.

H

HIPAA Security Rule Legislation that outlines the required administrative, technical, and physical safeguards to prevent unauthorized access to protected health care information.

I

ICD-9-CM Listing of codes for medical diagnoses; will eventually be replaced by ICD-10-CM.

Inpatient Refers to a patient admitted and discharged from a hospital with a length of stay of one or more days.

Insurance Aging report A report that shows an aging analysis of insurance accounts.

Insurance Collection reports Reports that are used to monitor outstanding claim balances of insurance carriers.

J

Journal Record of daily transactions listed in chronological order, also known as the book of original entry.

K

Knowledge base Searchable collection of updated information about a topic.

L

Ledger A group of accounts in which debits and credits are posted from the book of original entry.

M

Medicaid Health insurance offered by the government for low-income people (called MediCal in California).

Medicare Government health insurance made available to elderly and disabled people.

Medisoft Program Date The date used by the Medisoft program to process transactions. Unless specifically set, the program uses the current date stored by the computer.

Menu bar Listing of menus, from which options are selected, within a program.

Modifiers One- or two-digit codes that allow more-specific descriptions to be entered for the services the physician performed.

MultiLink code A code that incorporates a number of related procedure codes.

N

New patient A patient who has never visited the medical office or has not received professional care from any of the providers in the office in the last three years.

O

Once-a-month billing A patient billing system in which all statements are printed and mailed once a month, all at the same time.

Outpatient Refers to a patient who is treated for a medical condition at a facility but who does not stay a full twenty-four hours.

P

Patient Aging Applied Payment report Detailed report that shows an aging analysis of patient accounts.

Patient billing code A code that indicates the schedule of fees that applies to the patient.

Patient Collection report A report that is used to identify outstanding patient balances and monitor the collections process.

Patient information form A form completed by a patient that includes personal information such as name, address, employer, insurance coverage, and any known allergies.

Patient ledger Record of all activity (charges, payments, and adjustments) in an individual patient's account.

Patient Ledger report A report that lists the account activity for each patient for a specified time period and shows the current balance and any unpaid charges.

Patient statement A list of the amount of money a patient owes, organized by the amount of time the money has been owed, the procedures performed, and the dates the procedures were performed.

Payables Money owed by a practice but not yet sent to suppliers.

Payments Cash, checks, credit cards, or electronic funds transfers received for medical services rendered.

Practice Analysis report Detailed report that shows the practice's revenue for a period of time.

Procedure A service performed by a physician or other provider.

Providers The medical staff members, such as doctors and physical therapists, who perform the various services.

R

Receivables Money owed to a medical practice but not yet received from patients and insurance companies.

Remainder statements Statements that list only those charges that are not paid in full after all insurance carrier payments have been received.

Remittance advice (RA) A document received from an insurance carrier that lists patients, dates of service, charges, and the amount paid or denied.

Removable media device A device that stores data but is not a permanent part of a computer.

Restoring data The process of retrieving data from backup storage devices.

S

Signature on file Field used to indicate whether a patient's signature authorizing treatment and payment is on file.

Standard statements Statements that show all charges regardless of whether the insurance carrier has paid on the transactions.

T

Toolbar A bar located below the menu bar that provides an alternate method of accessing program options. Icons provide rapid access to program options.

Transactions Charges, payments, and adjustments for services provided to patients.

TRICARE A government health insurance plan for eligible dependents of military personnel.

Type Field used to identify an individual or another party as a patient or a guarantor.

Index

L

Ledger
  defined, 2
  general, 3
  patient. *See* Patient ledger; Patient
    ledger report
List Only option, 114
List reports
  described, 156
  viewing, 156–157
Locate (magnifying glass) button, 49

M

Manual systems
  claims, 18–21
  encounter forms (superbills),
    16–17
Medicaid
  described, 7
  Medicaid and TRICARE folder,
    72–74
Medical billing assistant
  day-to-day activities of, 3–16
  records kept by, 3–9
Medicare, described, 7
Medisoft
  adjustment transactions, 88,
    127–128
  backing up data files, 52–56, 82,
    104, 134, 158
  charge transactions, 88–97
  chart numbers, 46–47, 49
  claim management, 110–120
  Crystal Reports Preview window,
    144–145
  databases, 17, 48–50, 112
  dates in, 45, 91, 174, 176–180
  deleting d'ata, 44, 120
  editing data, 44–46, 81–82, 98–101,
    113, 119–120
  entering data, 8, 44–46, 76–82,
    88–104, 122–127
  exiting, 38, 53–54, 82, 104, 134, 158
  exporting files from, 144–145
  help options, 36–38, 48
  Knowledge Base, 38
  menu bar, 28–33, 34–35, 44
  menu navigation, 28–33, 34–35
  nature of, 28
  payment transactions, 8, 97–103,
    120–128
  printing in. *See* Printing in
    Medisoft
  Program Date, 35–36, 45, 174
  removing data disk, 38
  Report Designer, 157
  reports. *See* Reports in Medisoft
  restoring data files, 55–56
  saving data, 44, 94

searching in, 18–19, 48–50
  Standard Patient Lists option, 154
  starting, 34
  toolbar, 33–34
  viewing in, 54–55, 101, 144–145,
    156–157
  windows, 44–46. *See also specific*
    windows
Menu bar, Medisoft, 44
  illustrated, 28
  list of options, 29–33
  navigating menus, 28–33, 34–35
  using, 34–35
Miscellaneous folder, 72, 73
Modifiers
  defined, 91
  using, 102–103
MultiLink code
  defined, 92
  using, 102–103

N

Name/address folder, 64
New patient
  adding, 64–67, 76, 77–81
  defined, 62
  entering case data, 44–47, 76–82,
    88–104
  entering patient data, 76–82, 88–104

O

Office Hours, Medisoft, 173–182
  backing up data files, 182
  changing appointments, 180–181
  date of appointment, 176–180
  deleting appointments, 180–181
  entering, 175
  entering appointments, 175–176
  entering data, 175–176
  exiting, 175, 182
  New Appointment Entry dialog
    box, 175–176
  new patients, 180
  overview, 173–174
  previewing schedules, 181
  printing schedules, 181–182
  time of appointment, 176, 179
Once-a-month billing, 132–133
Online help, 37, 38
Other information folder, 65–66
Outpatient, defined, 91

P

Passwords, 18
Patient Aging Applied Payment
  report
  described, 147–148
  sample, 148

Patient billing, 27–38. *See also* Claim
  management; Medisoft
  computerized systems, 18–21
  day-to-day activities, 3–16
  defined, 3
  maintaining patient information,
    10, 82
  manual systems, 16–17
  overview of, 4
  records kept by medical billing
    assistant, 3–9
  simulation, 163–171
  steps in, 3–16
Patient Billing Code field, 66
Patient by Diagnosis report
  described, 154
  sample, 155
Patient/Case radio button, 76, 77
Patient Collection report
  described, 149
  sample, 150
Patient data files. *See* Data files
Patient day sheet, 140–145
  defined, 140
  printing, 142–145
  sample, 143
Patient/Guarantor window, 65
Patient Indicator field, 66
Patient information.
    See also Medisoft
  adding new patient, 64–67, 76,
    77–81
  basic, 10, 17
  in charge transactions, 88–97
  editing, 81–82
  entering case data, 44–47, 76–82,
    88–104
  entering patient data, 76–82,
    88–104
  maintaining, 10, 82
  organization of, 62–75
  patient/guarantor information
    requirements, 64–67
  in payment transactions,
    97–103
  searching, 48–49
  updating case data, 82
Patient information form
  defined, 62
  Medisoft database information, 10
  sample, 5, 63
Patient ledger, 14–16
  defined, 14
  entering payments on, 8
  manual preparation, 16–17
  sample, 15–16
Patient Ledger report, 151–154
  computerized preparation, 151–154
  described, 151
  printing, 153–154
  sample, 152